PEDIATRICS, CHILD AND ADOLESCENT HEALTH

ADOLESCENCE AND BEHAVIOR ISSUES IN A CHINESE CONTEXT

PEDIATRICS, CHILD AND ADOLESCENT HEALTH

SERIES EDITOR - JOAV MERRICK

NATIONAL INSTITUTE OF CHILD HEALTH AND HUMAN DEVELOPMENT,
MINISTRY OF SOCIAL AFFAIRS, JERUSALEM

Child and Adolescent Health Yearbook 2011
Joav Merrick (Editor)
2012. ISBN: 978-1-61942-782-2 (Hardcover)
2012. ISBN: 978-1-61942-783-9 (e-book)

Child and Adolescent Health Yearbook 2012
Joav Merrick (Editor)
2012. ISBN: 978-1-61942-788-4 (Hardcover)
2012. ISBN: 978-1-61942-789-1 (e-book)

Child Health and Human Development Yearbook 2011
Joav Merrick (Editor)
2012. ISBN: 978-1-61942-969-7 (Hardcover)
2012. ISBN: 978-1-61942-970-3 (e-book)

Child Health and Human Development Yearbook 2012
Joav Merrick (Editor)
2012. ISBN: 978-1-61942-978-9 (Hardcover)
2012. ISBN: 978-1-61942-979-6 (e-book)

Tropical Pediatrics: A Public Health Concern of International Proportions
Richard R Roach, Donald E Greydanus, Dilip R Patel, Douglas N Homnick and Joav Merrick (Editors)
2012. ISBN: 978-1-61942-831-7 (Hardcover)
2012. ISBN: 978-1-61942-840-9 (e-book)

Understanding Autism Spectrum Disorder: Current Research Aspects
Ditza A Zachor and Joav Merrick (Editors)
2012. ISBN: 978-1-62081-353-9 (Hardcover)
2012. ISBN: 978-1-62081-390-4 (e-book)

Developmental Issues in Chinese Adolescents
Daniel TL Shek, Rachel CF Sun and Joav Merrick (Editors)
2012. ISBN: 978-1-62081-262-4 (Hardcover)
2012. ISBN: 978-1-62081-270-9 (e-book)

Positive Youth Development: A New School Curriculum to Tackle Adolescent Developmental Issues
Hing Keung Ma, Daniel TL Shek and Joav Merrick (Editors)
2012. ISBN: 978-1-62081-384-3 (Hardcover)
2012. ISBN: 978-1-62081-385-0 (e-book)

Positive Youth Development: Theory, Research and Application
Daniel TL Shek, Rachel CF Sun and Joav Merrick (Editors)
2012. ISBN: 978-1-62081-305-8 (Hardcover)
2012. ISBN: 978-1-62081-347-8 (e-book)

Transition from Pediatric to Adult Medical Care
David Wood, John G Reiss, Maria E Ferris, Linda R Edwards and Joav Merrick (Editors)
2012. ISBN: 978-1-62081-409-3 (Hardcover)
2012. ISBN: 978-1-62081-412-3 (e-book)

PEDIATRICS, CHILD AND ADOLESCENT HEALTH

ADOLESCENCE AND BEHAVIOR ISSUES IN A CHINESE CONTEXT

DANIEL TL SHEK
RACHEL CF SUN
AND
JOAV MERRICK
EDITORS

nova publishers
New York

For permission to use material from this book please contact us:
Telephone 631-231-7269; Fax 631-231-8175
Web Site: http://www.novapublishers.com

Library of Congress Cataloging-in-Publication Data

Adolescence and behavior issues in a Chinese context / editors, Daniel T.L. Shek, Rachel C.F. Sun, and Joav Merrick (Health Services, Division for Intellectual and Developmental Disabilities, Ministry of Social Affairs and Social Services, Jerusalem, Israel, and others).

pages cm

Includes index.

ISBN: 978-1-62618-614-9 (hardcover)

1. Teenagers--China. 2. Adolescence--China. 3. Youth development--China. 4. Adolescent psychology--China. I. Shek, Daniel T. L. II. Sun, Rachel C. F. III. Merrick, Joav, 1950-

HQ799.C55A34 2013

305.2350951--dc23

2013013140

Published by Nova Science Publishers, Inc. † New York

Contents

INTRODUCTION: ADOLESCENCE AND BEHAVIOR ISSUES

Rachel CF Sun, Daniel TL Shek and Joav Merrick

There is co-morbid occurrence of adolescent problem behaviors, and these behaviors manifest differently and vary in severity (1). For instance, some adolescents who withdraw from stress and distress addict to substance and internet use (2,3), whereas some act out in the form of misbehavior and delinquency (4). In particular, research findings have shown that there are gender differences, with boys tend to employ externalizing and risk-taking behavior as ventilation, while girls tend to internalize stress and become depressed (5,6). Nevertheless, different problem behaviors may share similar etiologies (7). Adopting the ecological approach, adolescents' behaviors result from the complex interplay between themselves and the surrounding environment. Their engagement in problem behaviors, like substance abuse (8), internet addition (9), and depression and suicidal ideation (10), are fueled by various risk factors, together with inadequate protective factors, at the personal level and in their family, school, peers and community. Therefore, it is pertinent to depict the profiles, correlates and causes of different problem behaviors, for such a holistic understanding help developing corresponding remedies.

In preventive science, preventive and interventional remedies are the common means to tackle adolescent problem behaviors. However, it is argued that such prevention and intervention are dealing with manifest problems and thus not sufficient enough, unless there are simultaneous developmental and educational programs addressing the underlying needs of adolescents and strengthening their potentials to deal with their own issues and problems. In fact, there is a growing consensus that adolescents' problem behaviors could be reduced by promoting their thriving strengths (11) and psychosocial competencies (12,13). There are also research findings showing that positive youth development programs were related to reduction of problem behavior as well as healthy changes among adolescents in both Western contexts (14,15) and Chinese cultural contexts (16,17). Yet, programs aiming at promoting positive youth development and well-being, with demonstrated program effectiveness, are still sparse in various communities (18,19).

To further the inquiries of "what are the phenomena underlying adolescent problem behaviors?" and "what can be done to tackle the issue effectively?", more research studies are necessary to examine the socio-demographic and bio-psycho-social profiles related to problem behaviors. These studies can include samples at different developmental stages (i.e., not only adolescents, but also children and early adults), in various cultural contexts and communities, in order to generate a more comprehensive profile. Moreover, it is pertinent to understand the causes of problem behaviors holistically from multi-disciplinary perspectives. In addition to research studies investigating the concurrent relationships among the variables, longitudinal research is needed to trace the developmental directionality and trajectory of problem behaviors. Furthermore, it is of interest to explore the adolescents' perceptions and causal explanations of problem behaviors so as to unveil their underlying troubles and match up with their needs. All these provide insights for developing and implementing corresponding preventive and developmental programs as one of the effective strategies for maintaining adolescent well-being and reducing problem behaviors. At the same time, conducting rigorous program evaluation and quality assurance are indispensable for an effective program to facilitate positive changes among adolescents.

This book is a response to the concerns raised in the preceding paragraphs. There are chapters on the risk and protective factors on adolescent developmental issues in different parts of the world, particularly China and Hong Kong. We earnestly hope that these papers can give further insights on the nature of adolescent developmental issues and ways on how adolescent health can be promoted.

Assistant professor Rachel CF Sun, PhD
Faculty of Education,
The University of Hong Kong,
Pokfulam Road, Hong Kong, P.R. China
E-mail: rachels@hku.hk

Professor Daniel TL Shek, PhD, FHKPS, BBS, JP
Department of Applied Social Sciences,
The Hong Kong Polytechnic University,
Hunghom, Kowloon, Hong Kong, P.R. China
E-mail: ssdaniel@inet.polyu.edu.hk

Professor Joav Merrick, MD, MMedSci, DMSc
National Institute of Child Health and Human Development,
Division for Intellectual and Developmental Disabilities,
Ministry of Social Affairs,
Jerusalem , Israel
E-mail: jmerrick@zahav.net.il

REFERENCES

[1] Bryant AL, Schulenberg J, Bachman JG, O'Malley PM, Johnston LD. Understanding the links among school misbehavior, academic achievement, and cigarette use: a national panel study of adolescents. Prev Sci 2000;1:71-87.

[2] Hawkins JD, Catalano RF, Miller JY. Risk and protective factors for alcohol and other drug problems in adolescence and early adulthood: implications for substance abuse prevention. Psychol Bull 1992;112:64-105.

[3] Young KS. Internet addiction: symptoms, evaluation, and treatment. In: VandeCreek L, Jackson T, editors. Innovations in clinical practice: a source book Vol. 17. Sarasota, FL: Professional Resource Press, 1999:19-31.

[4] Weerman FM, Harland P, van der Laan PH. Misbehavior at school and delinquency elsewhere: a complex relationship. Crim Justice Rev 2007;2:358-79.

[5] Eme RF, Kavanaugh L. Sex differences in conduct disorder. J Clin Child Psychol 1995;24:406-26.

[6] Montague M, Cavendish W, Enders C, Dietz S. Interpersonal relationships and the development of behavior problems in adolescents in urban schools: a longitudinal study. J Youth Adolescence 2010;39:646-57.

[7] Shaffer HJ, LaPlante DA, LaBrie RA, Kidman RC, Donato AN, Stanton MV. Toward a syndrome model of addiction: multiple expressions, common etiology. Harvard Rev Psychiat 2004;12:367-74.

[8] Shek DTL. Tackling adolescent substance abuse in Hong Kong: where we should and should not go? TheScientificWorldJournal 2007;7:2021-30.

[9] Shek DTL, Sun RCF, Yu L. Internet addiction. In: Pfaff DW, editor. Neuroscience in the 21st century: basic and clinical. Amsterdam: Springer. In press.

[10] Sun RCF, Hui EKP. Building social support for adolescents with suicidal ideation: implications for school guidance and counselling. Brit J Guid Couns 2007;35:299-316.

[11] Lerner RM, von Eye A, Lerner JV, Lewin-Bizan S, Bowers EP. The meaning and measurement of thriving: a view of the issues. J Youth Adolescence 2010;39:707-19.

[12] Catalano RF, Hawkins JD, Berglund ML, Pollard JA, Arthur MW. Prevention science and positive youth development: competitive or cooperative frameworks? J Adolescent Health 2002;31:230-9.

[13] Sun RCF, Shek DTL. Life satisfaction, positive youth development, and problem behaviour among Chinese adolescents in Hong Kong. Soc Indic Res 2010;95:455-74.

[14] Jelicic H, Bobek DL, Phelps E, Lerner RM, Lerner JV. Using positive youth development to predict contribution and risk behaviors in early adolescence: findings from the first two waves of the 4-H study of positive youth development. Int J Behav Dev 2007;31:263-73.

[15] Lewin-Bizan S, Bowers EP, Lerner RM. One good thing leads to another: cascades of positive youth development among American adolescents. Dev Psychopathol 2010;22:759-70.

[16] Shek DTL, Sun RCF. Effectiveness of the Tier 1 Program of Project P.A.T.H.S.: findings based on three years of program implementation. TheScientificWorldJournal 2010;10:1509-19.

[17] Shek DTL, Yu L. Prevention of adolescent problem behavior: longitudinal impact of the Project P.A.T.H.S. in Hong Kong. TheScientificWorldJournal 2011;11:546-67.

[18] Shek DTL. Quality of life of Chinese people in a changing world. Soc Indic Res 2010;95:357-61.

[19] Shek DTL, Yu L. A review of validated youth prevention and positive youth development programmes in Asia. Inter J Adolesc Med Health. In press.

ADOLESCENT BEHAVIOR

In: Adolescence and Behavior Issues in a Chinese Context ISBN: 978-1-62618-614-9
Editors: DTL Shek, RCF Sun and Joav Merrick

Chapter 1

SCHOOL-BASED DRUG PREVENTION IN THE UNITED STATES: INSIGHTS FOR HONG KONG

***Shane S Wong*[1] *and Daniel TL Shek, PhD, FHKPS, BBS, JP*[2,3,4,5,6 *]**

[1]Stanford University School of Medicine, Stanford, CA, US
[2]Department of Applied Social Sciences, The Hong Kong Polytechnic University, Hong Kong, PRC
[3] Centre for Innovative Programmes for Adolescents and Families, Department of Applied Social Sciences, The Hong Kong Polytechnic University, Hong Kong, PRC
[4]Kiang Wu Nursing College of Macau, Macau, PRC
[5]Department of Social Work, East China Normal University, Shanghai, PRC
[6]Division of Adolescent Medicine, Department of Pediatrics, Kentucky Children's Hospital, University of Kentucky College of Medicine, Lexington, KY, US

ABSTRACT

This chapter reviews effective school-based drug prevention programs implemented in the United States. Research studies in major academic databases, policy review papers from academic and research institutes, and government reports from funding and administrative agencies relating to school-based drug prevention were reviewed. California and Washington states were used as examples to understand state-level efforts for drug prevention. Common principles of exemplar school-based drug prevention programs according to structure, content and delivery were summarized; relevant legislation and funding schemes that guide the implementation of such programs in the United States were identified. It is argued that effective program principles, legislation and funding schemes in the United States provide valuable lessons for determining future directions for drug prevention programs in Hong Kong.

* Correspondence: Professor Daniel T.L. Shek, PhD, FHKPS, BBS, JP, Chair Professor of Applied Social Sciences, Faculty of Health and Social Sciences, Department of Applied Social Sciences, The Hong Kong Polytechnic University, Room HJ407, Core H, Hunghom, Hong Kong. E-mail: daniel.shek@polyu.edu.hk.

INTRODUCTION

Because of its high social costs and growing severity in the global context, substance abuse has attracted much research attention from different disciplines, particularly in the area of substance abuse prevention. A review of the major databases shows that much research effort has been spent to understand substance abuse prevention. Literature searches up to March 2011 based on the search terms "substance abuse" and "prevention" showed that there were 3,066 citations in PsycINFO, 5,100 citations in CINAHL and 3,041 citations in MEDLINE. However, using "substance abuse", "prevention" and "Chinese" as the search terms, literature search showed that there were 5, 15 and 17 citations in PsycINFO, CINAHL and MEDLINE, respectively. Similarly, using "substance abuse", "prevention" and "Hong Kong" as the search terms, literature searches showed that there were 4, 4 and 4 citations in PsycINFO, CINAHL and MEDLINE, respectively. These figures clearly show that more research on substance abuse prevention should be conducted in different Chinese contexts, including Hong Kong.

We can use two "C"s to describe the characteristics of substance abuse in the global context. The first "C" is that there are *changing patterns* of substance abuse. In different countries, the types of substances commonly abused have been changed from heroin to psychotropic substances such as ecstasy and ketamine. In addition, abuse of synthetic drugs (e.g., tranquilizers) and drugs that can be bought over the counter (e.g., cough medicine) has become more popular. Regarding the second "C", although the manifestations of substance abuse vary across countries, there are many *commonalities* involved. For example, the figures on substance abuse have increased in both urban and rural areas of both under-developed and developed countries and such trends have attracted much public attention. With the rise of postmodern thoughts in which relativity in values is emphasized, more adolescents are abusing substances. Furthermore, substance abuse has been found to be associated with many other social problems, such as health hazards, family problems and crimes.

With specific reference to Hong Kong, there are several worrying observations regarding adolescent substance abuse (1,2). First, an examination of the substance abuse figures in the past twenty years showed that there were three peaks in the substance abusers figures reported to the Central Registry of Drug Abuse (CRDA) maintained by the Narcotics Division of the Government. The first peak was in mid-1990s, which was related to the abuse of depressants and tranquilizers. The second peak was in early 2000s and was closely related to ecstasy abuse. The third peak occurred in the past few years and was related to ketamine abuse. Second, statistics showed that there is a gradual decline in the age of first abuse of drugs among adolescents. Third, with the return of Hong Kong back to China in 1997, cross-border abuse has become an emergent problem in Hong Kong. Finally, the findings based on school surveys showed that substance abuse is a growing problem in the school context (3).

What strategies can be used to deal with the adolescent substance abuse problems? There are generally two approaches. The first strategy is supply reduction which is mainly carried out by law enforcement and legislation. Through this approach, it is expected that the supply of illicit drugs or drugs liable to abuse will decrease. Nevertheless, the sole reliance on supply reduction is not effective. The second approach is demand reduction, which is mainly carried out by publicity and preventive drug education. In this latter approach, focus is commonly put on the weakening of risk factors and strengthening of protective factors in adolescents with high risk for substance abuse.

In the United States, there has been a concerted emphasis in recent decades towards identifying and implementing effective youth drug prevention programs. School-based educational programs have been among the most popular preventive measures (4). Although it is intuitively appealing to conduct preventive drug education, it is important to know whether such education is really effective or not. In the literature on preventive drug education, there are numerous examples showing that programs based on good will and passion alone may not be effective programs. An example is the Project D.A.R.E. (Drug Abuse Resistance Education) Program, which was founded in 1983 in Los Angeles. The program has been implemented in 75% of the school districts in the U.S.A. and in more than 43 countries around the world to help young people stay away from drugs. Unfortunately, several longitudinal studies have repeatedly showed that the program did not work (5,6). As pointed out by Rosenbaum and Hanson, "...can this popular school-based program prevent drug use at the stages in adolescent development when drugs become available and are widely used, namely, during the high school years?" Unfortunately, the answer to the question is 'no' (7). Obviously, popularity and enthusiasm alone do not guarantee program success.

Against the above background, the present paper attempts to understand the implementation of preventive drug education programs in the United States with specific reference to three issues. First, using California and Washington states as examples, state mandates on the implementation of preventive drug education programs are examined. Second, federal and state funding policies are reviewed.

Finally, characteristics of effective preventive drug education programs and mechanisms for identifying such programs are reviewed. Based on the present review, the implications of the present review to preventive drug education in Hong Kong are explored.

OUR SEARCH

Related materials from different sources were reviewed in this study. First, research studies in major academic databases, including PsycINFO, CINAHL and MEDLINE with the search terms "substance abuse", "prevention", "United States" were reviewed. Second, policy review papers from non-profit organizations such as the Cochrane Collaboration and World Health Organization were reviewed. Third, government reports from funding and administrative agencies relating to school-based drug prevention such as the National Institute on Drug Abuse and the Substance Abuse and Mental Health Administration were reviewed. California and Washington State were used as examples to understand state-level efforts for drug prevention. Several questions are addressed in this review:

1. Is there any state mandate for implementation of drug prevention programs?
2. What federal funding is available for substance abuse prevention programs?
3. What state funding is available for substance abuse prevention programs?
4. What are the characteristics of effective substance abuse prevention programs?
5. How do schools identify effective substance abuse prevention programs?

WHAT WE FOUND

State mandates for drug prevention programs

In the United States, the National Health Education Standards are written expectations of the knowledge and skills that students should acquire to promote personal health, which provide a framework for states to develop a curriculum in health education (8).

Currently, drug prevention education is required in 38 of the 50 states (National Association of State Boards of Education, 2011). In the state of California, drug prevention education is required for all students from Grade 1 to Grade 12, as mandated by California Education Code (9). These Education Code mandates require instruction on the nature of drugs and their health effects in elementary and secondary schools, training and reevaluation of drug education teachers with approved programs, dissemination of model drug-prevention programs to schools, development of a model drug abuse prevention program for grades two, four and six, and development of a statewide system to improve program delivery, and give high priority to in-service training programs for school staff on drug abuse prevention.

In Washington State, drug prevention education is required for all students from Grade 1 through high school, as part of Health and Fitness education mandated by the Basic Education Act (10). The specific content for drug prevention education is outlined by the Health and Fitness Essential Academic Learning Requirements, with a Grade Level Expectation for every grade from Grade 1 to Grade 8 plus High School Health, which outlines the grade-specific concepts and skill that must be taught.

Federal funding for substance abuse prevention programs

Part A of Title IV 21st Century Schools, also known as the Safe and Drug-Free Schools and Communities Act (SDFSCA), is the United States federal government's primary initiative to prevent drug abuse, as well as violence, among school-aged children. It was first established by the 1986 Anti-Drug Abuse Act, and was most recently re-authorized and amended in 2002 by the No Child Left Behind Act (11). The funding program requires all schools receiving funds to implement programs to prevent illegal use of alcohol, tobacco, and drugs, involve parents and communities, and foster a safe and drug-free learning environment that supports student academic achievement.

Through the SDFSCA State Education Agency Grant program, state educational agencies are awarded non-competitive formula grants to create programs deterring drug abuse among elementary and secondary students, with at least 93 percent of funds required to be distributed to local education agencies (12). In fiscal year 2009, the program funded $228.8 million in grants to state education agencies, with the California Department of Education receiving $28.1 million, and the Washington Department of Public Instruction receiving $3.8 million (13). Local education agencies (e.g., school districts, charter schools) can then apply to their state education agency for funding, which will be approved if the proposed program meets the Principle of Effectiveness under Section 4115 of the SDFSCA, and awarded as non-competitive grants by formula based on number of low-income students and total student enrollment (14). Funds are allocated to school districts based on student enrollment at approximately $3.60 per student per school year (15). However, schools can opt not to apply for such funds. In fiscal year 2009/2010, funding was distributed to approximately 94% (793 of 846) of the school districts in California (16).

The SDFSCA administers another non-competitive formula grant to every state through the Governor's Grants program, which targets special need and underserved school-aged youth. Administered by a state agency designated by each state governor, these funds are further distributed as competitive discretionary grants to community-based and other nonprofit entities to support drug-prevention activities. In 2009, $57.3 million in total federal funding was disbursed through this program, with the California Department of Alcohol and Drug Programs receiving $7.0 million and the Washington Department of Community, Trade and Economic Development receiving $950,000 (13).

The SDFSCA also provides competitive discretionary funding directly to local education agencies and non-profit community programs. The Safe School/Healthy Students Grants program funds local education agencies to develop community-wide approaches to prevent drug abuse in coordination with community-based organizations. In 2009, $77.8 million was funded through the program, with California's 19 awardees receiving a combined $25.8 million and one Washington State local education agency receiving $1.5 million (13). The Mentoring Grants program also funds local education agencies and community-based organizations to promote school-based mentoring programs to prevent drug abuse. In 2009, $47.0 million was funded through the program, with California's 44 awardees receiving a combined $8.0 million and Washington State's 7 awardees receiving a combined $1.3 million (13). Finally, the School-Based Drug Testing program funds local education agencies and nonprofit entities to support school-based drug testing programs. These programs are limited to athletic programs, extracurricular competitive activities, and voluntary drug testing with written consent. In 2009, $6.9 million was funded through the program, with California's 3 awardees receiving a combined $250,000 and Washington State's 2 awardees receiving a combined $190,000 (13).

Apart from the SDFSCA, the other major source of federal funding for drug prevention originates from the Department of Health and Human Services' budget for the Substance Abuse and Mental Health Services Administration (17). SAMHSA's Substance Abuse Prevention and Treatment Block Grant provides non-competitive funding by formula to each state for drug abuse treatment and prevention. In fiscal year 2010, a total of $1.7 billion was granted, with California receiving $251 million and Washington State receiving $35 million (17). According to 2007 data, California used 22.8% of its Block Grant ($56.9 million of the $250 million) for primary prevention through the California Department of Alcohol and Drug Programs. The Department was also funded $11.6 million and $6.8 million from other federal funds and state funds respectively. During the same year, Washington State used 22.1% of its Block Grant to administer the Division of Alcohol and Substance Abuse's Prevention and Intervention Service, its primary program for drug prevention (18). In addition, the Division received $1.1 million from state funding for substance abuse prevention efforts.

SAMHSA also provides competitive discretionary funding through the Center for Substance Abuse Prevention. The Center administers several grant programs, including Drug Free Communities, Capacity Building Initiative, Ready-to-Respond Initiative, and the Strategic Prevention Framework State Incentive Grants programs (17). In fiscal year 2010, California awardees received $15.6 million in competitive discretionary funding for substance abuse prevention, while Washington awardees received $4.5 million.

State funding for drug prevention programs

In California, Healthy Start was established in 1991 through Senate Bill 620, the Healthy Start Support Services for Children Act, to improve student learning and support families (19). The California Department of Education administers Healthy Start and awards two-year Planning, five-year Operational, and seven-year Combined Planning and Operational competitive discretionary grants to local education agencies (LEAs). In its most recent year of funding, a total of $10 million was granted to 23 school districts (20). Between 1991 and 2007, more than 1 million students in 1,388 schools had been enrolled in the program (19).

Each local Healthy Start provides a system of comprehensive, school-integrated health, psychosocial, and educational services. The school-linked services initiative promotes the reconfiguration of existing community resources, and the center at or near the school site serves as the gateway for a continuum of services, such as youth development, health education or substance abuse prevention, for students and families who need assistance.

Another state source of funding is California's Department of Alcohol and Drug Programs, which was established upon enactment of the Health and Safety Code, Division 10.5, Sections 11750 (Stats. 1979, Ch. 679). It is designated as the Single State Agency (SSA) responsible for administering and coordinating the state's efforts in alcohol and drug abuse prevention, treatment, and recovery services. It has an annual budget of more than $600 million from both federal and state sources. In 2007, it spent $76.5 million on primary prevention programs, with $6.8 million originating from the non-competitive state funds (18).

In Washington State, state funding for drug prevention programs is provided by the Department of Community, Trade and Economic Development (DCTED), the Department of Social and Health Services (DSHS), and the Family Policy Council (15).

Between 1999-2001, the DCTED funded $90,000 towards the Governor's Council on Substance Abuse, which researches alternatives for state policy action, works with government agencies and communities to develop goals, and advises the governor on substance abuse policy and programs. The DCTED also funds the the Community Mobilization against Substance Abuse and Violence program, which provides competitive discretionary grants for local communities to develop and implement strategies to reduce the demand and supply of illegal drugs (21). In 2009, $840,000 in state funding was provided for the program.

The Washington Department of Social and Health Services (DSHS) administers formula funding through the Division of Alcohol and Substance Abuse to the Office of the Superintendent of Public Instruction for school-based programs that prevent chemical dependency. In 2008, $970,000 from the state general fund was granted (21).

The Prevention and Intervention Services Programs is Washington's primary school-based drug and alcohol abuse prevention and early intervention program (15). This program was originally created as part of the 1989 Omnibus Alcohol and Controlled Substance Act of the Washington State Legislature, and strives to prevent the drug abuse and assist students to overcome problems of substance abuse.Over two-thirds of middle and high school students are estimated to participate in the services program, with over 20,000 students being served every year (22).

Finally, the Family Policy Council was established in 1992 to work with the Community Public Health and Safety Networks, a network of community-based, volunteer boards that provides communities autonomy, resources, and opportunities to recommend policy change to address seven youth risk behavior areas, including the youth substance abuse (15). In 2008, they received $2.2 million in state funding (21).

Overall, it is estimated that California provides $16.8 million annually from state funds for drug prevention programs, in addition to $153.3 million from federal funds. The state of Washington provides an estimated $4.1 million annually from state funds for primary drug prevention, in addition to $19.9 million from federal funds. With enrollment figures at 6.2 million students in California and 1.0 million students in Washington, approximately $27.4 per California student and $24.0 per Washington student is spent annually on drug prevention programs.

Choice of drug prevention programs

Since 2002, the Safe and Drug-Free Schools and Communities Act (SDSFCA) has required that all drug prevention programs funded by the program meet the Principle of Effectiveness: that all programs be grounded in scientifically based research (14).

The Office of Safe and Drug-Free Schools recommends the use of the National Registry of Evidence-Based Programs and Practices (NREPP) and FindYouthInfo Program Directory to identify effective prevention programs. The NREPP rates programs based on the quality of the research supporting intervention outcomes and the quality and availability of training and implementation materials (23). FindYouthInfo Program Directory rates programs using four dimensions of effectiveness: conceptual framework, program fidelity, evaluation design, and empirical evidence (24).

In California, the majority of programs implemented are listed in these registries (16). Similarly, funding from the Washington State Division of Alcohol and Substance Abuse's Prevention and Intervention Service requires that a minimum of 50% of funded programs be evidence-based, while innovative programs must follow principles of effectiveness in their design (25).

Exemplar model drug prevention programs

Based on the recommendations from the National Institute of Drug Abuse (26), ratings from SAMHSA's National Registry of Evidence-Based Programs and Practices, ratings from FindYouthInfo Program Directory, and the relative popularity of SDFSCA-funded prevention programs implemented in California, the following is a list of general principles for effective programs, and five exemplar model drug prevention programs in the United States.

Effective school-based drug prevention program principles: Structure

The principles concerning program structure describe how effective school-based drug prevention programs are organized and constructed.

1. Programs should be research-based (27).
2. Program curriculum should span multiple grades and developmental periods with age-appropriate curriculum (28). First, prevention programs can be designed to intervene as early as preschool to address risk factors for drug abuse, such as aggressive behavior, poor social skills, and academic difficulties (29). Second, prevention programs for elementary school children should target improving academic and social-emotional learning to address risk factors for drug abuse, such as early aggression, academic failure, and school dropout. Education should focus on the following skills (30): self-control; emotional awareness; communication; social problem-solving; and academic support, especially in reading. Finally, prevention programs for middle or junior high and high school students should increase academic and social competence with the following skills (31,32): study habits and academic support; communication; peer relationships; self-efficacy and assertiveness; drug resistance skills; reinforcement of antidrug attitudes; and strengthening of personal commitments against drug abuse.
3. Prevention programs should be long-term with repeated interventions (i.e., booster programs) over a number of years to reinforce the original prevention (4). Research shows that the benefits from middle school prevention programs diminish without follow-up programs in high school (32), and programs that include refresher sessions are more effective (33). Prevention programs should include sufficient follow-up (27).
4. Teacher training and support should be part of prevention programs (27). Training should include good classroom management practices, such as rewarding appropriate student behavior, which foster students' positive behavior (30). In particular, interactive programs are more difficult to teach and facilitate, and require teachers with specialized teaching and classroom management skills (27, 34). If teachers are uncomfortable or untrained in interactive techniques, they are unlikely to implement such programs effectively (27).
5. The structure and philosophy of the programs should encourage broad-based involvement in decision making related to their organizational structure (28).
6. Prevention programs should include features that promote their sustainability (28).

Effective school-based drug prevention program principles: Content

The principles concerning program content describe the information, skills and strategies that are taught.

1. Prevention programs should enhance protective factors and reverse or reduce risk factors that are related to the initiation and maintenance of substance abuse (28,35).
2. Prevention programs should address all forms of drug abuse, alone or in combination, including the underage use of legal drugs (e.g., tobacco or alcohol); the use of illegal drugs (e.g., marijuana or heroin); and the inappropriate use of legally obtained substances (e.g., inhalants), prescription medications, or over-the-counter drugs (36). Programs should address the validity of the gateway hypothesis and thus include alcohol and tobacco prevention (28).

3. Programs which develop individual social skills are one of the most effective forms of school-level intervention for the prevention of the early drug use (37). Programs that are built upon social-influence models are recommended (33).
4. Comprehensive health education is an important component for effective curriculum (27). Complementary general health and life skills programs appear to produce greater change than skill-based education programs alone, suggesting that drug prevention education is best integrated within a well-founded health curriculum (4).
5. Normative education, as an important mediator for drug use, is an important component of an effective curriculum (27,38).
6. Inclusion of substance-specific knowledge, such as information about short-term and long-term negative consequences, as a component of the program, is a determining factor for effectiveness (33).

Effective school-based drug prevention program principles: Delivery

The principles concerning program delivery describe the adaptation, implementation and evaluation of the program.

1. Prevention programs should address the type of drug abuse problem in the local community (35).
2. Programs must be provided at a developmentally appropriate time and particularly when interventions are most likely to have an impact on behavior to be effective. These include periods when most students are experiencing initial exposure to drugs, or key transition points such as transition to secondary school (26-28). The skills and knowledge provided need to be developmentally relevant to the students, need to be applicable to their life experiences, and need to be of immediate practical use to them (39).
3. Prevention programs should be tailored to address risks specific to population or audience characteristics, such as gender and ethnicity, to improve program effectiveness (40). The program should also be socioculturally sensitive (27,28).
4. When communities adapt programs to match their needs, community norms, or differing cultural requirements, they should retain core elements of the original research-based intervention (41).
5. Prevention programs are most effective when they employ interactive techniques that promote active participation of program providers and recipients, such as role-playing, active modeling, and discussion (31). Such programs are at a minimum twice as effective as non-interactive program and up to four times as effective as non-interactive programs (42,43). Programs should expend a meaningful degree of resources in engaging the target population (28).
6. Prevention programs should include an evaluation component (27).

DISCUSSION

The implementation of preventive drug education programs in the United States is reviewed in this paper. Three observations can be highlighted from this review. First, with specific reference to California and Washington states, there are state mandates on the implementation of drug prevention programs in school contexts. In other words, schools in these two states are required to carry out preventive drug education in a compulsory manner. Second, there is federal as well as state funding for the implementation of preventive drug education. Third, there are effective preventive drug education programs and there are databases on such programs. Furthermore, there is a quest for effective programs and there are criteria for judging whether a program is effective or not.

What are the implications of the present review to preventive drug education in Hong Kong? In Hong Kong, preventive drug education has several features. First, although topics on drug abuse are included in the curriculum frameworks of different subjects (e.g., General Studies in primary schools), there is no definitive curriculum and designated time. Second, under the healthy school policy, although schools are expected to carry out preventive drug education, it is up to the school to decide which format will be used. Actually, many schools use morning assemblies and stand-alone drug talks as preventive drug education programs. Third, with very few exceptions (e.g., 44-45), validated preventive drug education programs are almost non-existent in Hong Kong. Fourth, teachers know very little about substance abuse in pre-service training courses.

There are several implications of the present review to preventive drug education in Hong Kong. First, in view of the growing severity of adolescent drug abuse problem in Hong Kong, there is a need to consider whether drug education should be carried out in a mandatory manner. One argument that is commonly put forward against this proposal is that it violates human rights. In fact, this is a very weak argument if we observe that preventive drug education is carried out in states of California and Washington in the United States, a country that places heavy emphasis on human rights. Furthermore, if drug prevention is really important, then it should be seriously considered in the policy making process.

The second implication is on the issue of funding. In the present context, there is no resource specifically earmarked for preventive drug education in the school context. Schools have to either use their own resources or to apply for external funding to run preventive education programs. Although the Hong Kong Government has recently injected an additional amount of HK$3 billion to the Beat Drugs Fund, many anti-drug programs, including publicity and preventive drug education, treatment and rehabilitation and research are supported by the fund. Obviously, the federal and state funding arrangements can serve as interesting reference for Hong Kong to learn. The third implication is on the characteristics of effective programs. Several observations on the effective preventive education program can be highlighted from the review.

In the first place, it is important to note that there are useful guidelines for evaluating the qualities of effective preventive drug education programs. Second, it is noteworthy that there are databases containing effective and scientifically credible preventive drug education programs. Third, the review shows that evaluation is very important in the development of effective preventive drug education programs.

Table 1. Summary of federal funding for drug prevention programs

Federal Funding Source	Federal Funding Program	Annual Federal Funding	State Administration Agency	Grantees	Funding Received for Primary Prevention	Prevention Program Requirements
Safe and Drug-Free Schools and Communities Act	State Education Agency Grants (Non-competitive formula funding to every state education agency; non-competitive formula funding to local education agency applicants)	$232.1 million (2009)	Department of Education (CA)	Local education agencies	$28.1 million (2009)	At least 93 % of funds distributed to local education agencies, with applications approved if proposed prevention program meets the Principle of Effectiveness.
			Office of the Superintendent of Public Instruction (WA)	Local education agencies	$3.8 million (2009) (Plus $970,000 from state funds)	
	Governor's Grants (Noncompetitive formula funding to every state; competitive discretionary funding to local applicants)	$57.3 million (2009)	Department of Alcohol & Drug Programs (CA)	County Alcohol & Other Drug office program services	$7.0 million (2009)	Targets special need and underserved school-aged youth
			Department of Community, Trade & Economic Development, Community Mobilization Program (WA)	Counties, education systems, and community-based non-profit entities (300 programs in 37 communities)	$950,000 (2009)	
	Safe School/Healthy Students Grants (Competitive discretionary funding)	$77.8 million (2009)		19 awardees (CA)	$25.8 million (2009)	Awarded to local education agencies coordinating with community-wide organizations
				1 awardee (WA)	$1.5 million (2009)	
	Mentoring Grants (Competitive discretionary funding)	$47.0 million (2009)		44 awardees (CA)	$8.0 million (2009)	Awarded to local education agencies and community- based organizations
				7 awardees (WA)	$1.3 million (2009)	

Table 1. (Continued)

Federal Funding Source	Federal Funding Program	Annual Federal Funding	State Administration Agency	Grantees	Funding Received for Primary Prevention	Prevention Program Requirements
	School-Based Drug Testing (Competitive discretionary funding)	$6.9 million (2009)		3 awardees (CA)	$250,0000 (2009)	Limited to athletic programs, extracurricular competitive activities, and voluntary drug testing with written consent
				2 awardees (WA)	$190,000 (2009)	
Department of Health and Human Services: Substance Abuse and Mental Health Administration	Substance Abuse Prevention and Treatment Block Grant (Non-competitive formula funding)	$1.7 billion (2010)		Department of Alcohol and Drug Programs (CA)	$56.9 million (2007) (Plus $11.6 million from other federal funds, and $6.8 from state funds)	Includes all primary prevention programs, including school-based programs
				Division of Alcohol and Substance Abuse's Prevention and Intervention Service (WA)	$7.7 million (2007) (Plus $1.1 million from state funds)	
	Center for Substance Abuse Prevention (Competitive discretionary funding)	$86.7 million (2010)		Multiple awardees (CA)	$15.6 (2010)	Discretionary funding programs include Strategic Prevention Framework State Incentive Grant Program, Drug-Free Communities, Ready-To- Respond Initiative, and Capacity Building Initiative.
				Multiple awardees (WA)	$4.5 million (2010)	
Total		$2.2 billion			$153.3 million (CA) $19.9 million (WA)	

Table 2. Summary of state funding for drug prevention programs

State	State Funding Source	Administration Agency	Annual Funding	Prevention Program Requirements
California	Healthy Start (Competitive discretionary funding)	Department of Education	$10 million (2007)	Distributed to high-need school districts, country offices of education, or charter schools on a competitive basis to develop comprehensive school-integrated system of health, psychosocial, and educational services. Grantees must provide a 25 percent match of funds.
	Health and Safety Code (Non-competitive funding)	Department of Alcohol and Drug Programs	$6.8 million (2007) (Plus $68.5 million from federal funds)	
Washington	Department of Community, Trade & Economic Development	Community Mobilization Against Substance Abuse and Violence (Competitive discretionary funding)	$840,000 (2008) (Plus $950,000 from federal funds)	Provides competitive grants to communities that use the Communities That Care (CTC) model to promote positive development and prevent substance abuse.
		Governor's Council on Substance Abuse (Non-competitive funding)	$45,000 (2001)	Researches policy, collaborates with government and communities to develop goals, and advises the governor on substance abuse policy and programs.
	Department of Social and Health Services, Division of Alcohol and Substance Abuse (Non-competitive formula funding)	Office of the Superintendent of Public Instruction	$970,000 (2008) (Plus $3.8 million from federal funds)	Funds school-based Prevention and Intervention Services Programs, which target alcohol and drug abuse.
	Family Policy Council (Competitive discretionary funding)	Community Public Health and Safety Networks	$2.2 million (2009)	Funds 42 networks of community-based, volunteer boards to address seven youth risk behavior areas.
Total			$16.8 million (CA) $4.1 million (WA)	

Table 3. Details of five exemplar model drug prevention programs

	Program Type	Audience	Information	Skills	Theory	Methods	Duration
Botvin's Life Skills Training	Universal (designed for the general population, such as all students in a grade)	Elementary to high school	Normative Drug influences	Drug resistance Self-management Social skills Resilience Navigating developmental tasks	Social influence model Competence enhancement model	Facilitated discussion Role-playing scenarios Structured small-group activities	22.5 hours total Over 3 years
Project ALERT	Universal	Middle and high school	Nondrug norms Drug use consequences Benefits of non-use Prodrug pressures	Reasons not to use, Resisting prodrug pressures	Social influence model	Participatory activities Small-group activities Question-and-answer sessions Role-playing Rehearsal of skills Videos	10 hours total Over 2 years
Project Towards No Drug Use	Indicated (alternative schools or high-risk students	High school	Correct cognitive misperceptions	Motivation Self-control Decision-making Communication	Motivation-skills–decision-making model	Group discussions Games Role-playing exercises Videos Student worksheets	9 hours total
Too Good for Drugs	Universal	Kindergarten to grade 8 curriculum High school curriculum	Negative consequences of drug use Benefits of drug-free lifestyle Positive peer norms	Resisting peer pressure Goal-setting Decision-making Social bonding Self-respect Social skills Communication Managing emotions	Social Development Strategy Social Learning Theory	Role-playing Modeling Practicing and modeling skills Games	5-10 hours/ K-8 grade 3.5 hours/ high school grade
Second Step	Universal	Kindergarten to 5th grade curriculum Middle school curriculum	Normative education	Empathy Impulse control Anger management Positive goal-setting Decision-making	Cognitive behavioral intervention models Social learning theory Social information-processing theories	Group decision-making Modeling Coaching Practicing interpersonal situations Video or photo scenarios	17 hours / K-5 grade 9 hours/ middle school grade

The above observations have several important implications for preventive drug education in Hong Kong. First, professionals working in the field of substance abuse prevention (such as teachers and social workers) should understand that there are clear guidelines for differentiating effective programs from ineffective programs. Such understanding can help professionals to choose effective programs for adolescent clients. Second, there is an urgent need to establish databases on effective substance abuse programs in Hong Kong. It is noteworthy that there is currently no such databases in Hong Kong, not just in the area of substance abuse, but in other fields of human services as well. Finally, the review suggests that there is a need to promote the professional competence of workers in the field of preventive drug education. As suggested by Shek, Lam and Tsoi, evidence-based practice is just beginning in Hong Kong (46). Shek similarly pointed out this problem in evidence-based practice in human services in Hong Kong (47).

ACKNOWLEDGMENTS

This manuscript was supported by a Stanford University Medical Scholars Program grant to Shane Shucheng Wong. The contents of this article are solely the responsibility of the authors and do not necessarily represent the official views of the funding agencies. This chapter is based upon a paper published in the International Journal on Disability and Human Development (Wong SS, Shek DTL. School-based drug prevention in the United States: Insights for Hong Kong. Int J Disabil Hum Dev 2012;11(2):91-101). Permission has been obtained from the publisher to publish this modified version of the paper in this book.

REFERENCES

[1] Shek DTL. Tackling adolescent substance abuse in Hong Kong: where we should and should not go. ScientificWorldJournal 2007;7:2021–30.

[2] Shek DTL. School drug testing: a critical review of the literature. ScientificWorldJournal 2010;10:356–65.

[3] The 2008/09 survey of drug use among students [Internet]. Hong Kong: Narcotics Division, Security Bureau; c2009 - [updated 2002 Feb 25; cited 2011 Apr 2]. Available from: http://www.nd. gov. hk /en /survey_of_drug_use.htm

[4] Hawks D, Scott K, McBride N, Jones P, Stockwell T. Prevention of psychoactive substance use: a selected review of what works in the area of prevention. Geneva: World Health Organization, 2002.

[5] Ennett ST, Tobler NS, Ringwalt CL, Flewelling RL. How effective is drug resistance education? A meta-analysis of Project DARE outcome evaluations. Am J Public Health 1994;84:1394–401.

[6] West SL, O'Neil KK. Project DARE outcome effectiveness revisited. Am J Public Health 2004;94:1027–29.

[7] Rosenbaum DP, Hanson GS. Assessing the effects of school-based drug education: a six-year multilevel analysis of Project D.A.R.E. J Res Crime Delin 1998;35:381–412.

[8] Joint Committee on National Health Education Standards. National health education standards: achieving excellence. 2nd ed. Atlanta: American Cancer Society, 2007.

[9] State School Healthy Policy Database: Alcohol, Tobacco, and Drug Use Education [Internet]. Arlington (VA): National Association of State Boards of Education. c1998-[cited 2011 Mar 15]. Available from: http://nasbe.org/healthy_schools/hs/bytopics.php

[10] Office of Superintendent of Public Instruction. Health and fitness standards: essential academic learning requirements: a recommended grade-by-grade sequence for grade level expectations – grades K-12. Olympia: Office of Superintendent of Public Instruction, 2008.
[11] Noble PV. Safe and drug free schools. New York: Novinka Books, 2002.
[12] Office of Communications and Outreach. Guide to U.S. Department of Education programs: fiscal year 2010. Washington: U.S. Department of Education, 2010.
[13] Grant Award Database [Internet].Washington (DC): U.S. Department of Education. c2008 - [updated 2011 Feb 28; cited 2011 Apr 2]. Available from: http://wdcrobcolp01.ed.gov/CFAPPS/grantaward/start.cfm
[14] Office of Safe and Drug-Free Schools. Safe and drug-free school and communities act: non-regulatory draft guidance for state and local implementation of programs. Washington: U.S. Department of Education, 2004.
[15] Gookin K, Aos S. How much money does Washington State government spend on prevention programs for youth? Olympia: Washington State Institute for Public Policy, 2001 Jan. Document ID: 01-01-1201.
[16] Safe and Healthy Kids Program Office. Safe and Healthy Kids annual report: 2008-09 annual report summary for California. Washington: U.S. Department of Education, 2010.
[17] Substance Abuse and Mental Health Services Administration. SAMHSA grant awards - state summaries, formula and discretionary grant allotments FY 2010/2011. Washington: U.S. Department of Health & Human Services, 2010.
[18] Substance Abuse and Mental Health Services Administration. 2010 state snapshots: substance prevention and treatment programs. Washington: U.S. Department of Health & Human Services, 2010.
[19] California Department of Education. Health framework for California public schools kindergarten through grade twelve. Sacramento: California Department of Education, 2003.
[20] State schools chief Jack O'Connell announces recipients of $10 million in healthy start grants [Internet]. Washington: California Department of Education; c2007 – [cited 2011 Apr 2]. Available from: http://www.cde.ca.gov/nr/ne/yr07/yr07rel86.asp
[21] Office of Financial Management. DSHS - alcohol and substance abuse: recommendation summary. Olympia: Washington State Department of Social and Health Services, 2009.
[22] Deck DD. Addressing adolescent substance abuse: an evaluation of Washington's prevention and intervention services program: 2001–03 final report. Olympia: Office of Superintendent of Public Instruction, 2004.
[23] National Registry of Evidence-based Programs and Practices [Internet]. Washington (DC): U.S. Department of Health and Human Services. c2006 - [updated 2011 Jan 12; cited 2011 Mar 2]. Available from: http://nrepp.samhsa.gov/NREPPNews.aspx
[24] Background and methodology [Internet]. Washington: FindYouthInfo; c2010 - [cited 2011 Mar 16]. Available from: http://www.findyouthinfo.gov/
[25] Substance abuse prevention services [Internet]. Olympia: Washington State Department of Social and Health Services; c2011 - [cited 2011 Apr 2] Available from: http://www.dshs.wa.gov/dbhr/dapreventionservices.shtml
[26] Robertson EB, David SL, Rao SA. Preventing drug use among children and adolescents: a research based guide for parents, educators, and community leaders. Washington: National Institute on Drug Abuse, 2003.
[27] Dusenbury L, Falco M. Eleven components of effective drug abuse prevention curricula. J Sch Health 1995;65:420-5.
[28] Winters KC, Fawkes T, Fahnhorst T, Botzet A, August G. A synthesis review of exemplary drug abuse prevention programs in the United States. J Subst Abuse Treat 2007;32:371-80.
[29] Webster-Stratton C, Reid J, Hammond M. Preventing conduct problems, promoting social competence: a parent and teacher training partnership in Head Start. J Clin Child Psychol 2001;30:283–302.

[30] Ialongo N, Poduska J, Werthamer L, Kellam S. The distal impact of two first-grade preventive interventions on conduct problems and disorder in early adolescence. J Emot Behav Disord 2001;9:146–60.
[31] Botvin G, Baker E, Dusenbury L, Botvin E, Diaz T. Long-term follow-up results of a randomized drug-abuse prevention trial in a white middle class population. JAMA 1995;273:1106–12.
[32] Scheier L, Botvin G, Diaz T, Griffin K. Social skills, competence, and drug refusal efficacy as predictors of adolescent alcohol use. J Drug Educ 1999;29:251–78.
[33] Buehler A, Kroeger C. Report on the prevention of substance abuse. Cologne: Federal Centre for Health Education BZgA, 2006.
[34] Lloyd C, Joyce R, Hurry J, Aston M. The effectiveness of primary school drug education. Drugs Educ Prev Pol 2000;72:109–26.
[35] Hawkins JD, Catalano RF, Arthur M. Promoting science-based prevention in communities. Addict Behav 2002;90:951-76.
[36] Johnston LD, O'Malley PM, Bachman JG. Monitoring the Future national survey results on drug use, 1975–2002. Volume 1: Secondary School Students. Bethesda: National Institute on Drug Abuse, 2002.
[37] Faggiano F, Vigna-Taglianti F, Versino E, Zambon A, Borraccino A, Lemma P. School-based prevention for illicit drugs' use. Cochrane Database Syst Rev 2005;2:CD003020.
[38] Cuijpers P. Effective ingredients of school-based drug prevention programs: a systematic review. Addict Behav 2002;27:1009–23.
[39] McBride N, Midford R, Farringdon F, Phillips M. Early results from a school alcohol harm minimisation study: the school health and alcohol harm reduction project. Addiction 2000;95:1021-42.
[40] Oetting E, Edwards R, Kelly K, Beauvais F. Risk and protective factors for drug use among rural American youth. In: Robertson EB, Sloboda Z et al, eds. Rural substance abuse: state of knowledge and issues. Washington: National Institute of Drug Abuse, 1997:90–130.
[41] Spoth RL, Redmond D, Trudeau L, Shin C. Longitudinal substance initiation outcomes for a universal preventive intervention combining family and school programs. Psychol Addict Behav 2002;16: 129–34.
[42] Tobler N. Meta analysis of adolescent drug prevention programmes: results of the 1993 meta analysis. In: Bukoski W, ed. Meta analysis of drug abuse prevention programmes. Washington: National Institute on Drug Abuse, 1997:5-68.
[43] Tobler N, Stratton H. Effectiveness of school based drug prevention programs: a meta-analysis of the research. J Prim Prev 1997;18:71-128.
[44] Shek DTL, Ng CSM, Tsui PF. Qualitative evaluation of the project P.A.T.H.S.: findings based on focus groups. Int J Disabil Hum Dev 2010;9:307-13.
[45] Shek DTL, Ng CSM. Early identification of adolescents with greater psychosocial needs: an evaluation of the project P.A.T.H.S. in Hong Kong. Int J Disabil Hum Dev 2010;9: 291-9.
[46] Shek DTL, Lam MC, Tsoi KW. Evidence-based social work practice in Hong Kong. In: Thyer B, Kazi M, eds. International perspectives on evidence-based practice in social work. London: Venture Press, 2004:213-22.
[47] Shek DTL. Enthusiasm-based or evidence-based charities: personal reflections based on the Project P.A.T.H.S. in Hong Kong. ScientificWorldJournal 2008;8:802-10.

In: Adolescence and Behavior Issues in a Chinese Context ISBN: 978-1-62618-614-9
Editors: DTL Shek, RCF Sun and Joav Merrick

Chapter 2

PERCEIVED PARENTAL BEHAVIORAL CONTROL AND PSYCHOLOGICAL CONTROL IN CHINESE ADOLESCENTS IN SHANGHAI

***Xiao Y Han, PhD*[1]**
***and Daniel TL Shek, PhD, FHKPS, BBS, JP*[*,1,2,3,4,5]**
[1]Department of Social Work, School of Social Development,
East China Normal University, Shanghai, PRC
[2]Department of Applied Social Sciences,
The Hong Kong Polytechnic University, Hong Kong, PRC
[3]Centre for Innovative Programmes for Adolescents and Families,
The Hong Kong Polytechnic University, Hong Kong, PRC
[4]Kiang Wu Nursing College of Macau, Macau, PRC
[5]Division of Adolescent Medicine, Department of Pediatrics,
Kentucky Children's Hospital, University of Kentucky College of Medicine,
Lexington, KY, US

ABSTRACT

Chinese secondary school students in Shanghai (N = 3,022) responded to instruments measuring their subjective evaluation of parental behavioral control (including dimensions of parental knowledge, expectation, monitoring, discipline, and demandingness) and parental psychological control. Concerning the inter-relationships among different dimensions of parental behavioral control, different indicators of parental behavioral control were inter-related and parental monitoring was the strongest predictor of parental knowledge. Different aspects of parental behavioral control were differentially related to parental psychological control. Results also showed that paternal behavioral control was perceived to be significantly lower than maternal behavioral

* Correspondence: Professor Daniel T.L. Shek, PhD, FHKPS, BBS, JP, Chair Professor of Applied Social Sciences, Faculty of Health and Social Sciences, Department of Applied Social Sciences, The Hong Kong Polytechnic University, Room HJ407, Core H, Hunghom, Hong Kong. E-mail: daniel.shek@polyu.edu.hk.

control in terms of different indicators of behavioral control. The theoretical and practical implications of the present findings are discussed.

INTRODUCTION

In the literature on parenting, two types of parental control have been identified. The first type of parental control is behavioral control. According to Smetana and Daddis (1), behavioral control refers to "rules, regulations and restrictions that parents have for their children" (p. 563). In the model of parenting proposed by Maccoby and Martin (2), behavioral control or demandingness is an important dimension on which parenting can be assessed. The second type of parental control is psychological control that refers to "parents' attempt to control the child's activities in ways that negatively affect the child's psychological world and thereby undermines the child's psychological development" (p. 563). Barber (3) further pointed out that psychological control is a "neglected construct" in parenting and that "there is little research specifically measuring psychological control and its covariates" (p. 3313). With specific reference to the Chinese culture, it would be interesting to study both types of parental control because Chinese parents are commonly regarded as controlling.

Parental behavioral control has been commonly conceptualized in terms of parental monitoring (1,4), which refers to surveillance and/or tracking and whether the parent takes initiative to understand the child (5). However, parental monitoring is usually measured in terms of parental knowledge of children's activities, i.e., how much the parent knows about the situation of the child (6,7). Methodologically speaking, parental monitoring (i.e., surveillance) is different from parental knowledge of children's activities because parental knowledge does not necessarily involve monitoring activities and that children's voluntary disclosure of information is crucial. Besides, there is a need to recognize the multi-dimensional nature of parental behavioral control (i.e., parental attempt to control and mange the child's behavior) and to differentiate parental monitoring and parental knowledge of children's activities (1). An integration of the existing research findings shows that at least five different aspects of parental behavioral control should be differentiated: 1) parental knowledge, 2) parental expectations (i.e., parental rules and expectations towards children), 3) parental monitoring, 4) parental discipline (reward and punishment of the child in relation to parental expectations), and 5) global parental control with reference to some of the existing models of parenting, such as parental demandingness (2).

There are several questions that should be asked with reference to the construct of parental behavioral control. First, because few family studies have examined the inter-relationships among different dimensions of parental behavioral control (8,9), it is important to ask whether and how different dimensions of parental behavioral control are inter-correlated. In particular, although parental monitoring has commonly been operationalized in terms of parental knowledge, the relationship between the two domains has rarely been examined in the literature. Besides, it would be interesting to ask whether those parents who set high expectations about the children really track or monitor the related behavior of their children. Despite the limited research findings showing that parental monitoring (operationalized in terms of parental knowledge) was related to parental control (7,10), the overall picture is still not clear. Theoretically, it is expected that there should be correlation amongst different aspects of parental control.

Second, it would be theoretically and practically important to ask how different aspects of parental behavioral control (expectations, monitoring, discipline and demandingess) may predict parental knowledge. If parental knowledge is a valid indicator of parental monitoring, it was expected that relative to other aspects of parental behavioral control, parental monitoring would have the strongest relationship with parental knowledge. On the other hand, if the common criticism that parental knowledge is a poor indicator of parental monitoring, then parental monitoring would not be very predictive of parental knowledge.

Third, it would be interesting to ask whether parental behavioral control is related to parental psychological control. An examination of the related studies shows that while parental monitoring (operationalized in terms of parental knowledge) was negatively related to parental psychological control (1,4), the relationship was not stable across time (1). For example, Bean, Bush, McKenry and Wilson (11) found a significant positive relationship between parents' behavioral control and psychological control among African Americans but not in European Americans. In Galambos, Barker and Almeida's study (12), no significant relationship was found between the two types of parental control. Therefore, there is a need to further examine the relationship between parental behavioral control and psychological control, particularly with respect to different dimensions of parental behavioral control.

Finally, in view of the research findings that there were parental differences (fathers vs. mothers) in global parenting processes (13,14) and psychological control (8,9), it would be interesting to ask whether parental differences also exist in the multi-dimensional parental behavioral control. With particular reference to the Chinese culture, differential parenting styles for fathers and mothers are commonly reflected in the popular saying of "strict father, kind mother" (i.e., fathers exert more parental behavioral control than mothers, while mothers express more affection than fathers). Hence, it would be important to see whether Chinese fathers actually exert greater behavioral control than do the Chinese mothers as implicit in traditional Chinese beliefs (i.e., prediction based on traditional Chinese beliefs). On the other hand, as contemporary Chinese mothers are more involved in the socialization process (13,14), it would be predicted that parental behavioral control would be higher in Chinese mothers than in Chinese fathers.

In the context of Hong Kong, based on a sample of 3,017 Chinese secondary school students, Shek found that parental behavioral control can be regarded as a multi-dimensional construct and that different dimensions were inter-related with parental monitoring being the strongest predictor of parental knowledge. Although the relationship between parental psychological control and a composite indicator of parental behavioral control was weak, different dimensions of parental behavioral control were found to be related to parental psychological control in different ways (8). While the findings of Shek's study (8) are pioneer in this field, there is a need to know whether these results can be replicated in other Chinese contexts with relatively different cultural and societal characteristics. As such, the present study was conducted in Shanghai, a typical large city in China Mainland, to further examine the research questions stated above. Basically, four questions are examined in this study: 1) what are the inter-relationships amongst different aspects of behavioral control? 2) How do parental expectations, monitoring, discipline and demandingness predict parental knowledge? 3) What are the relationships between different aspects of parental behavioral control and psychological control? 4) Are there parental differences in parental behavioral control and psychological control?

OUR STUDY

A total of 3,022 junior secondary school students (1,512 males and 1,480 females with a mean age of 13.41 years) participated in the study. They were all Grade 6 and Grade 7 students recruited from 17 schools randomly selected from all secondary schools in Shanghai. The purpose of the study was mentioned and the confidentiality of the data collected was repeatedly emphasized to all of the students in attendance on the day of testing. The students were asked to indicate their wish if they did not want to participate in the study (i.e., "passive" informed consent was obtained from the students). All participants responded en masse to the questionnaire in a self-administration format. Adequate time was provided for the subjects to complete the questionnaire. A trained research assistant was present throughout the test administration process.

Instruments

The assessment tools employed in this study were developed by Shek (8,9). Several measures of parental control were used in this study as follows:

Paternal Knowledge Scale (PKNO) and Maternal Knowledge Scale (MKNO): Based on a review of the literature, seven items were developed to form the Paternal Knowledge Scale (Cronbach's alpha = 0.76). Identical items were used to assess maternal knowledge that formed the Maternal Knowledge Scale (Cronbach's alpha = 0.79). The total score of the items in each scale was used as an indicator of the level of parental knowledge of the child's behavior, with a higher score indicating a higher level of knowledge (8,9).

Paternal Expectation Scale (PEXP) and Maternal Expectation Scale (MEXP): Based on the literature, seven items were developed to form the Paternal Expectation Scale (Cronbach's alpha = 0.66). Identical items were used to assess maternal expectation that formed the Maternal Expectation Scale (Cronbach's alpha = 0.64). The total score of the items in each scale was used as an indicator of the level of parental expectation of the child's behavior, with a higher score indicating a higher level of expectation and requirement (8,9).

Paternal Monitoring Scale (PMON) and Maternal Monitoring Scale (MMON): Based on the literature, seven items were developed to form the Paternal Monitoring Scale (Cronbach's alpha = 0.78). Identical items were used to assess maternal monitoring that formed the Maternal Monitoring Scale (Cronbach's alpha = 0.76). The total score of the items in each scale was used as an indicator of the level of parental monitoring of the child's behavior, with a higher score indicating a higher level of monitoring (8,9).

Paternal Discipline Scale (PDIS) and Maternal Discipline Scale (MDIS): Based on the literature, five items were developed to form the Paternal Discipline Scale (Cronbach's alpha = 0.63). Identical items were used to assess maternal discipline that formed the Maternal Discipline Scale (Cronbach's alpha = 0.68). The total score of the items in each scale was used as an indicator of the level of reasonable parental discipline, with a higher score indicating a higher level of reasonable parental discipline of the child (8,9).

Paternal Parenting Style Scale and Maternal Parenting Style Scale: To assess global parental control with reference to the existing models on parenting, the Paternal Parenting Style Scale and Maternal Parenting Scale (15) were used. These two scales were developed to measure adolescents' self-perceived parenting practices, based on the framework of Maccoby and Martin (2). Shek further found that there were two stable dimensions in the scales: responsiveness and demandingness, based on which a modified version of the scales was developed (16). In this study, the Responsiveness Scale (13 items) and Demandingness Scale (7 items) developed by Shek were used (16), and showed satisfying reliability. The Cronbach's alphas for the Paternal Responsiveness Scale (PRES), Paternal Demandingness Scale (PDEM), Maternal Resonsiveness Scale (MRES), and Maternal Demandingness Scale (MDEM) were 0.76, 0.74, 0.76, and 0.75, respectively. The total score of each scale was used as an indicator of the level of parental responsiveness or demandingness, with a higher score indicating more positive parental attributes (8,9).

Paternal Psychological Control Scale (PPSY) and Maternal Psychological Control Scale (MPSY): Based on the literature (3,17), 10 items were developed to form the Paternal Psychological Control Scale (Cronbach's alpha = 0.88). Identical items were used to assess maternal psychological control that formed the Maternal Psychological Control Scale (Cronbach's alpha = 0.90). The total score of the items in each scale was used as an indicator of the level of parental psychological control, with a higher score indicating a higher level of control. Shek (18) showed that the scale possessed acceptable psychometric properties.

During the study, the adolescent participants were also requested to respond to other scales measuring different areas of psychological well-being. These include the Chinese version of the Hopelessness Scale, Mastery Scale, Life Satisfaction Scale, and Self-Esteem Scale (8,9). As the focus of this study was on parental behavioral and psychological control, results and psychometric properties of these scales are not reported in the present paper.

OUR FINDINGS

Inter-correlations among different dimensions of parental behavioral control were first calculated by Pearson correlation analysis and are presented in Table 1. To guard against Type 1 error, a multi-stage Bonferroni correction procedure was used (19). There are two observations that can be highlighted from the findings. First, different dimensions of parental behavioral control were all positively correlated, with correlation coefficients ranging from 0.12 to 0.61 indicating slight to modest strength of relationship. Second, the magnitude and pattern of correlation coefficients were similar across the paternal and maternal variables.

To examine the relative contribution of different dimensions of parental behavioral control to parental knowledge, multiple regression analyses were carried out for the paternal and maternal variables separately. Parental knowledge was used as the dependent variable and the other four dimensions of parental behavioral control were entered simultaneously as the independent variables. The results are shown in Table 2. Both analyses showed that parental expectation, monitoring and demandingness positively predicted parental knowledge, with parental monitoring being the strongest predictor. However, parental discipline did not predict parental knowledge (see Table 2).

Table 1. Inter-relationships among different measures of parental behavioral control

	PKNO/ MKNO	PEXP/ MEXP	PMON/ MMON	PDIS/ MDIS	PDEM/ MDEM
PKNO/MKNO	-	.42*	.60*	.23*	.46*
PEXP/MEXP	.39*	-	.55*	.41*	.41*
PMON/MMON	.61*	.53*	-	.34*	.46*
PDIS/MDIS	.23*	.38*	.34*	-	.22*
PDEM/MDEM	.39*	.32*	.39*	.14*	-

Note: Correlation coefficients for the paternal behavioral control variables are above diagonal. Correlation coefficients for the maternal behavioral control variables are below diagonal. PKNO: Paternal Knowledge Scale. PEXP: Paternal Expectation Scale. PMON: Paternal Monitoring Scale. PDIS: Paternal Discipline Scale. PDEM: Paternal Demandingness Scale. MKNO: Maternal Knowledge Scale. MEXP: Maternal Expectation Scale. MMON: Maternal Monitoring Scale. MDIS: Maternal Discipline Scale. MDEM: Maternal Demandingness Scale. A two-tailed multistage Bonferroni procedure was used to obtain the data related to all 20 correlations (19). *pFW* is based on the familywise Type 1 error rate. *pT* is the Type 1 error rate per test.

* pFW < .001 pT < .00005.

Table 2. Relationships between parental expectation, monitoring, discipline and demandingness (predictors) and paternal knowledge (criterion measure)

Dependent Variables	Predictor Variables	Beta	R^2
Paternal Knowledge (PKNO)	PEXP	.07*	.41
	PMON	.46*	
	PDIS	.00	
	PDEM	.23*	
Maternal Knowledge (MKNO)	MEXP	.07*	.40
	MMON	.50*	
	MDIS	.01*	
	MDEM	.17*	

Note: PKNO: Paternal Knowledge Scale. PEXP: Paternal Expectation Scale. PMON: Paternal Monitoring Scale. PDIS: Paternal Discipline Scale. PDEM: Paternal Demandingness Scale. MKNO: Maternal Knowledge Scale. MEXP: Maternal Expectation Scale. MMON: Maternal Monitoring Scale. MDIS: Maternal Discipline Scale. MDEM: Maternal Demandingness Scale. * p < .001.

The relationships between different dimensions of parental behavioral control and psychological control were examined through correlation analyses and the results are presented in Table 3. There are two observations that deserve attention. First, the magnitude of the related correlation coefficients was generally small (ranging from 0.02 to -0.18). Second, different dimensions of parental behavioral control were associated with psychological control in different directions: while parental knowledge and parental demandingness were negatively related to psychological control, parental expectation and discipline was positively related to psychological control. Third, the relationship between parental monitoring and psychological control was only significant for mothers at a borderline level and was non-significant for fathers.

Table 3. Relationships between parental behavioral control and parental psychological control

Variable	PPSY	Variable	MPSY
PKNO	-.18***	MKNO	-.12***
PEXP	.15***	MEXP	.21***
PMON	.02	MMON	.05[a]
PDIS	.27***	MDIS	.30***
PDEM	-.07***	MDEM	-.05[a]

Note: PKNO: Paternal Knowledge Scale. PEXP: Paternal Expectation Scale. PMON: Paternal Monitoring Scale. PDIS: Paternal Discipline Scale. PDEM: Paternal Demandingness Scale. PPSY: Paternal Psychological Control Scale. MKNO: Maternal Knowledge Scale. MEXP: Maternal Expectation Scale. MMON: Maternal Monitoring Scale. MDIS: Maternal Discipline Scale. MDEM: Maternal Demandingness Scale. MPSY: Maternal Psychological Control Scale. A two-tailed multistage Bonferroni procedure was used to obtain the data related to all 12 correlations (19). pFW is based on the familywise Type 1 error rate. pT is the Type 1 error rate per test.

[*] pFW < .05 pT < .005.

[a] Borderline significance; pT < .05.

Finally, regarding parental differences in behavioral control, a series of paired t-test with Bonferroni correction of the alpha level were performed. Consistent with our expectations, maternal control was stronger than paternal control in terms of parental knowledge, parental expectations, parental discipline and parental demandingness. However, no parental differences in psychological control were observed (Table 4).

Table 4. Paternal differences in behavioral control and psychological control

Paternal Variable	Mean	Maternal Variable	Mean	t value	Effect Size (Cohen's d)
PKNO	20.79	MKNO	21.81	-13.63***	0.26
PEXP	20.63	MEXP	20.92	-4.95***	0.09
PMON	18.71	MMON	20.45	-22.05***	0.41
PDIS	14.89	MDIS	15.38	-10.27***	0.18
PDEM	11.19	MDEM	12.16	-18.54***	0.27
PPSY	20.62	MPSY	20.73	-0.98	-

Note: PKNO: Paternal Knowledge Scale. PEXP: Paternal Expectation Scale. PMON: Paternal Monitoring Scale. PDIS: Paternal Discipline Scale. PDEM: Paternal Demandingness Scale. PPSY: Paternal Psychological Control Scale. MKNO: Maternal Knowledge Scale. MEXP: Maternal Expectation Scale. MMON: Maternal Monitoring Scale. MDIS: Maternal Discipline Scale. MDEM: Maternal Demandingness Scale. MPSY: Maternal Psychological Control Scale.

[*] p < .0001 (Bonferroni corrected alpha level = .05/6 = .008).

DISCUSSION

Consistent with our predictions and previous findings in Hong Kong (8,9), there were positive and moderate relationships among different dimensions of parental behavioral control. These findings indicate that the five scales all measure different aspects of parental behavioral control and thus provide some support for the convergent validity of the measures. In particular, with reference to the criticism that parental monitoring should not be operationalized in terms of parental knowledge, the significant relationship between parental knowledge and parental monitoring (Table 1) and the observation that parental monitoring was the strongest predictor of parental knowledge (Table 2) suggest that it may be legitimate to use parental knowledge as a measure of parental monitoring. Although there are doubts on whether parental knowledge is a valid indicator of parental behavioral control, the present findings showed that parental knowledge has a close relationship with other aspects of parental behavioral control. In the context of family assessment, there are two advantages of assessing parental knowledge. First, as compared to parental expectations and monitoring, it can be argued that assessment of parental knowledge is relatively easier in both parents and adolescent children because it is less intrusive. Second, information on parental knowledge also provides some hints of parental understanding of the situation of the child, which is often used as a treatment goal in family related intervention programs.

Regarding the relationship between parental behavioral control and psychological control, the present findings generally suggest that the relationship between behavioral control and psychological control is domain specific. Consistent with previous findings (1,4), parental knowledge and demandingness were found to be negatively related to parental psychological control. However, parental expectation and parental discipline were positively associated with parental psychological control. Because "there is little research specifically measuring psychological control and its covariates" [(3), p. 3313], the present findings are interesting additions to the literature. In future, more studies should be conducted to examine the relationships between these two domains particularly using indigenous concepts of parental control.

The weak relationship between parental behavioral control and parental psychological control found in the present study indicates that the two domains may be dissociated. The findings suggest that those who want to psychologically control their children may not really make enough efforts to monitor/manage their children on the behavioral level. There are two possible explanations for this dissociation. First, parents who are high in psychological control may not realize the importance of controlling their children behaviorally and/or they do not know how to control their children on the behavioral level. The second possible explanation is that as psychological control impairs the parent-child relationship, deterioration in the parent-child relationship would make behavioral control less possible. Another interesting aspect of the finding is that parental discipline was positively related to psychological control. This finding suggests that for psychologically controlling parents (i.e., controlling parents), they also tend to punish their children more.

Finally, the present study showed that Chinese adolescents perceived paternal behavioral control as lower than maternal behavioral control. As far as parental knowledge is concerned, maternal knowledge was perceived to be higher than paternal knowledge. With reference to parental expectations, monitoring, discipline and demandingness, fathers were consistently perceived as having lower scores than mothers across these dimensions. However, no parental differences were found for parental psychological control. The present study clearly demonstrates that paternal parental control is different from maternal control, irrespective of which indicator is used. According to Shek (20,21), the relatively higher maternal behavior control may be explained in terms of the relatively higher level of involvement of mothers in the socialization process. Since there is no related study in China Mainland, the present study can be regarded as pioneering.

The present findings challenge the popular Chinese belief of "strict father, kind mother" held by Chinese people while concur with Shek's argument (22) that this popular belief has been changed to "kind fathers, strict mothers". Furthermore, as Chinese mothers are commonly blamed for the problem behavior in their children (as exemplified in the Chinese belief of "ci mu dor bai er" – a kind mother spoils the child), the present observation that mothers were more involved in behavioral control than did the fathers can help to demystify such popular myths and empower the mothers. As Caplan (23) pointed out, "blaming mothers for their children's psychological problems has a long and, unfortunately, respected history, particularly among mental health professionals" (p. 70). In a review of the portrait of fathers and mothers in the literature, Caplan and Hall-Corquodale (24) also showed that mothers were commonly described in negative terms and they were blamed for causing a wide range of childhood psychopathology. With reference to paternal and maternal behavioral control processes, the present findings clearly pointed out that Chinese fathers were less involved than did the mothers, which may lead to problem behavior in adolescents.

There are several limitations of this study. First, because the assessment of parental control was based on self-report measures from the perspective of the child, there might be bias involved. The inclusion of observational data in real life settings based on the "outsiders" and inclusion of informants from different perspectives would give a more complete picture as far as assessment of the related processes is concerned. Second, because the sample was recruited from Chinese adolescents in Shanghai, there is a need to replicate the findings in different cultural contexts, including those based on Chinese Americans. Finally, because the present study is a cross-sectional study, the causal relationships among the different domains are not clear. Obviously, longitudinal studies play an indispensable role in clarifying the inter-relationships amongst the different processes of parental behavioral control and the linkage between behavioral control and psychological control further (21,22).

As far as intervention is concerned, Chinese parents in mainland China should be helped to understand the nature of parental behavioral and psychological control and the ways to strengthen behavioral control but not psychological control (8,9). Besides, adolescents should also be educated about family processes and how family dynamics will affect adolescent development. It is noteworthy that such programs are grossly lacking in the Chinese literature (25). One notable exception is the Project P.A.T.H.S. where bonding (i.e., links with significant others and family bondage) is included in the program. While the evaluation of the Project P.A.T.H.S. is very encouraging (26-30), there is a need to develop more positive youth development programs with family focus in different Chinese communities.

ACKNOWLEDGMENTS

The preparation for this paper and the study were financially supported by the Wofoo Foundation. This chapter is based upon a paper published in the International Journal on Disability and Human Development (Han XY, Shek DTL. Perceived parental behavioral control and psychological control in Chinese adolescents in Shanghai. Int J Disabil Hum Dev

2012;11(2):107-12). Permission has been obtained from the publisher to publish this modified version of the paper in this book.

REFERENCES

[1] Smetana JG, Daddis C. Domain-specific antecedents of parental psychological control and monitoring: the role of parenting beliefs and practices. Child Dev 2002;73:563-80.

[2] Maccoby EE, Martin JA. Socialization in the context of the family: parent-child interaction. In: Mussen PH (Series ed.), Hetherington EM (Vol.ed), Handbook of child psychology, vol. 4, Socialization, personality, and social development. New York: Wiley, 1983:1-100.

[3] Barber BK. Parental psychological control: revisiting a neglected construct. Child Dev 1996;67:3296-319.

[4] Pettit GS, Laird RD, Dodge KA, Bates JE, Criss MM. Antecedents and behavior-problem outcomes of parental monitoring and psychological control in early adolescence. Child Dev 2001;72:583-98.

[5] Dishion TJ, McMahon RJ. Parental monitoring and the prevention of child and adolescent problem behavior: a conceptual and empirical formulation. Clin Child Fam Psychol Rev 1998;1:61-75.

[6] Crouter AC, Head MR. Parental monitoring and knowledge of children. In Bornstein MH, editor. Handbook of parenting, vol. 3. Mahwah, NJ: L Erlbaum Assoc, 2002:461-483.

[7] Kerr M, Stattin H. What parents know, how they know it, and several forms of adolescent adjustment: further support for a reinterpretation of monitoring. Dev Psychol 2000;36:366-80.

[8] Shek DTL. Perceived parental behavioral and psychological control in Chinese adolescents in Hong Kong. Am J Fam Ther 2006a;34:163-76.

[9] Shek DTL. Perceived parent-child relational qualities and parental behavioral and psychological control in Chinese adolescents in Hong Kong. Adolescence 2006b;41:563-81.

[10] Stattin H, Kerr M. Parental monitoring: a reinterpretation. Child Dev 2000;71:1072-85.

[11] Bean RA, Bush KR, McKenry PC, Wilson SM. The impact of parental support, behavioral control, and psychological control on the academic achievement and self-esteem of African American and European American adolescents. J Adolesc Res 2003;18:523-41.

[12] Galambos NL, Barker ET, Almeida DM. Parents do matter: trajectories of change in externalizing and internalizing problems in early adolescence. Child Dev 2003;74:578-94.

[13] Shek DTL. Adolescents' perceptions of paternal and maternal parenting styles in a Chinese context. J Psychol 1998;132:527-37.

[14] Shek DTL. Chinese adolescents' perceptions of parental differences in parenting characteristics, parent-adolescent communication and parent-adolescent relationship. Adolescence 2000;35:135-46.

[15] Lamborn SD, Mounts NS, Steinberg L, Dornbusch SM. Patterns of competence and adjustment among adolescents from authoritative, authoritarian, indulgent, and neglectful families. Child Dev 1991;62:1049-65.

[16] Shek DTL. Parenting characteristics and adolescent psychological well-being: a longitudinal study in a Chinese context. Genet Soc Gen Psychol Monogr 1999;125:27-44.

[17] Barber BK,editor. Intrusive parenting: how psychological control affects children and adolescents. Washington, DC: American Psychological Association, 2002.

[18] Shek DTL. Assessment of perceived parental psychological control in Chinese adolescents in Hong Kong. Res Soc Work Pract 2006c;16(4):382-91.

[19] Larzelere RE, Mulaik SA. Single-sample tests for many correlations. Psychol Bull 1977;84:557-69.

[20] Shek DTL. Perceived parental control and parent-child relational qualities in Chinese adolescents in Hong Kong. Sex Roles 2005;53(9-10):635-46.

[21] Shek DTL. A longitudinal study of perceived differences in parental control and parent-child relational qualities in Chinese adolescents in Hong Kong. J Adolesc Res 2007;22(2):156-88.

[22] Shek DTL. Economic disadvantage, perceived family life quality, and emotional well-being in Chinese adolescents: a longitudinal study. Soc Indic Res 2008;85(2):169-89.

[23] Caplan PJ. Take the blame off mother. Psychol Today 1986;20:70-1.

[24] Caplan PJ, Hall-McCorquodale I. Mother-blaming in major clinical journals. Am J Orthopsychiatry 1985;55:345-53.
[25] Shek DTL, Yu L. A review of validated youth prevention and positive youth development programmes in Asia. Int J Adolesc Med Health 2011;23:317-24.
[26] Shek DTL, Sun RCF. Effectiveness of the Tier 1 Program of Project P.A.T.H.S.: findings based on three years of program implementation. Sci World J 2010;10:1509-19.
[27] Shek DTL, Ma CMS. Impact of the Project P.A.T.H.S. in the junior secondary school years: individual growth curve analyses. Sci World J 2011;11:253-66.
[28] Shek DTL, Yu L. Prevention of adolescent problem behavior: longitudinal impact of the Project P.A.T.H.S. in Hong Kong. Sci World J 2011;11:546-67.
[29] Shek DTL, Ng CSM, Tsui PF. Qualitative evaluation of the Project P.A.T.H.S.: findings based on focus groups. Int J Disabil Hum Dev 2010;9(4):307-14.
[30] Shek DTL, Ng CSM. Early identification of adolescents with greater psychosocial needs: an evaluation of the Project P.A.T.H.S. in Hong Kong. Int J Disabil Hum Dev 2010;9(4):291-300.

In: Adolescence and Behavior Issues in a Chinese Context
Editors: DTL Shek, RCF Sun and Joav Merrick
ISBN: 978-1-62618-614-9

Chapter 3

SOCIO-DEMOGRAPHIC AND FAMILY CORRELATES OF HOPELESSNESS AMONGST ADOLESCENTS IN SHANGHAI, CHINA

Xiao Y Han, PhD[1]
and Daniel TL Shek, PhD, FHKPS, BBS, JP[*,1,2,3,4,5]
[1]Department of Social Work, School of Social Development, East China Normal University, Shanghai, PRC
[2]Department of Applied Social Sciences, The Hong Kong Polytechnic University, Hong Kong, PRC
[3]Centre for Innovative Programmes for Adolescents and Families, The Hong Kong Polytechnic University, Hong Kong, PRC
[4]Kiang Wu Nursing College of Macau, Macau, PRC
[5]Division of Adolescent Medicine, Department of Pediatrics, Kentucky Children's Hospital, University of Kentucky, College of Medicine, Lexington, KY, US

ABSTRACT

Chinese secondary school students (n=3,022) responded to measures of adolescent hopelessness, perceived parental behavioral control, parental psychological control, and parent-child relational qualities. Results showed that roughly one-fifth of Chinese adolescents displayed signs of hopelessness. Adolescent hopelessness was positively related to age and boys displayed a lower level of hopelessness than did girls. Adolescent hopelessness was also related to parental education, marital status of the parents, and economic disadvantage. While parental behavioral control was negatively related to adolescent hopelessness, parental psychological control was positively associated with adolescent hopelessness. Adolescents who perceived parent-child relational qualities to

[*] Correspondence: Professor Daniel T.L. Shek, PhD, FHKPS, BBS, JP, Chair Professor of Applied Social Sciences, Faculty of Health and Social Sciences, Department of Applied Social Sciences, The Hong Kong Polytechnic University, Room HJ407, Core H, Hunghom, Hong Kong, PRC. E-mail: daniel.shek@polyu.edu.hk.

be better showed a lower level of hopelessness. Parental psychological control and parental trust emerged to be two important predictors of adolescent hopelessness in Chinese adolescents.

Introduction

Although there are different views on the concept of spirituality and different components have been proposed, presence or loss of hope is commonly regarded as an important component of spirituality (1). For example, Highfield and Cason (2) proposed that there are four types of spiritual needs, including need for meaning and purpose in life, need to receive love, need to give love, and need for hope and creativity. Thompson (3) outlined five types of spiritual distress, including spiritual pain, spiritual alienation, spiritual guilt, spiritual loss, and spiritual despair (loss of hope). Similarly, Anandarajah and Hight (4) suggested that hope and its sources should be assessed. In the therapeutic context, it is common to set "inducement of hope" as a therapeutic goal. Empirically, there are research findings showing that hopelessness was positively related to adolescent mental health, such as depressive symptoms (5) and suicidal ideations (6). In a process model assessing adolescent suicide risk for suicide, Stoelb and Chiriboga (7) argued that hopelessness was a primary factor determining an adolescent's level of or risk for suicide.

Despite the importance of hope or hopelessness in adolescent adjustment, there are several limitations intrinsic to the existing studies of adolescent hopelessness. First, our understanding of socio-demographic correlates of adolescent hopelessness is grossly inadequate. Research findings on the relationships between hopelessness and age, gender, parental education, parental marital status, and economic disadvantage are also not conclusive (8). Besides, there are few studies investigating hopelessness among young people experiencing economic disadvantage. Obviously, studies of demographic correlates of adolescent hopelessness would enable helping professionals to identify high-risk adolescents in terms of hopelessness at an early stage.

Second, few studies have to date examined the relationships between parental control processes, including behavioral control and psychological control, and adolescent hopelessness. Regarding parental behavioral control, an integration of the existing research findings (9) suggests that at least five different aspects of parental behavioral control (i.e., parental attempt to control and mange the child's behavior) should be differentiated, including parental knowledge (i.e., how much the parent knows about the situation of the child), parental expectations (i.e., parental rules and expectations of the parent), parental monitoring (i.e., parental surveillance and tracking and whether the parent takes initiative to understand the child), parental discipline (reward and punishment of the child in relation to parental expectations), and global parental demandingness. Garber and Flynn (10) showed that psychological control was positively related to adolescent hopelessness but behavioral control was not related to adolescent hopelessness. As different dimensions of parental control may be related to adolescent hopelessness in a different manner, it would be interesting to look at the relationships between different aspects of parental control and adolescent hopelessness.

Third, the relationship between parent-child relational qualities and hopelessness is unclear (11). Besides, it would be interesting to know whether different aspects of parent-child relational qualities, such as mutual trust between the parents and adolescent children, were related to adolescent hopelessness. In fact, mutual trust between parents and adolescent children is grossly neglected in the literature (12). In this study, mutual trust between parents and adolescents, children's readiness to communicate with the parents, and children's satisfaction with parental control were included as indicators of parent-child relational qualities.

Finally, although studies have been conducted to examine hopelessness in the West, few studies have examined adolescents' quality of life such as hopelessness in Chinese adolescents (13, 14). A survey of the literature showed that hopelessness was related to pathological symptoms (15) and was identified as an important predictor of suicidal ideation (16, 17). On the other hand, hopelessness was negatively related to positive mental health measures, including purpose in life, self-esteem, life satisfaction, and existential well-being (1). However, few scientific studies have been conducted in mainland China. Also, with a few exceptions, no studies have employed large and representative samples to examine adolescent hopelessness.

Four research questions are addressed in this chapter as follows:

1. What is the pattern of hopelessness among Chinese adolescents in Shanghai?
2. What are the socio-demographic correlates (including age, gender, parental education, parental marital status, and economic disadvantage) of hopelessness among Chinese adolescents in Shanghai? Based on previous studies (8), it was expected that: a) age would be positively related to hopelessness; b) boys would display a higher level of hopelessness than girls; and c) parental education would be negatively related to adolescent hopelessness. Based on previous studies (8), it was also expected that adolescents in non-intact families would show a higher level of hopelessness than adolescents in intact families. Finally, it was predicted that adolescents experiencing economic disadvantage would have a higher level of hopelessness than adolescents without economic disadvantage (8).
3. What are the relationships between perceived parental behavioral control processes (indexed by parental knowledge, expectation, monitoring, discipline, and global parental control based on Western literature), psychological control, and adolescent hopelessness? Based on the literature (8), it was predicted that there would be a negative relationship between parental behavioral control and hopelessness and a positive relationship between parental psychological control and hopelessness.
4. What is the relationship between parent-child relational qualities (child's satisfaction of parental control, readiness of the child to communicate, parental trust of the child, and child's trust of the parent) and adolescent hopelessness? Based on the literature (8), it was predicted that there would be a negative relationship between parent-child relational qualities and hopelessness.

OUR STUDY

A total of 3,022 junior secondary school students (1,512 males and 1,480 females with a mean age of 13.41 years) participated in the study. They were all Grade 6 and Grade 7 students recruited from 17 schools randomly selected from all secondary schools in Shanghai. The purpose of the study was mentioned and confidentiality of the data collected was repeatedly emphasized to all of the students in attendance on the day of testing. The students were asked to indicate their wish if they did not want to participate in the study (i.e., "passive" informed consent was obtained from the students). All participants responded en masse to the questionnaire in a self-administration format. Adequate time was provided for the participants to complete the questionnaire. A trained research assistant was present throughout the test administration process.

Instruments

The assessment tools employed in this study were developed by Shek (8, 9). The measures are outlined below:

Assessment of Adolescent Hopelessness: Adolescent hopelessness was assessed by the Chinese Hopelessness Scale in this study. The Hopelessness Scale was devised by Beck, Weissman, Lester and Trexler (18) to measure the sense of hope in an individual. The Chinese Hopelessness Scale was developed by Shek (19) who reported that the scale was valid and reliable. Based on factor analysis, Shek (19) showed that three factors (Hopelessness, Certainty about the Future, and Future Expectation) were abstracted from the scale. In the present study, items based on the Hopelessness sub-scale of the scale (10 items) were used to assess hopelessness (alpha=0.88; mean inter-item correlation=0.43).

Assessment of Parental Control: Different aspects of behavioral control (including parental knowledge, expectations, monitoring, discipline, and global parental control) and psychological control were assessed as follows:

1. *Paternal Knowledge Scale (PKNO) and Maternal Knowledge Scale (MKNO):* Seven items were developed to form the Paternal Knowledge Scale (e.g., "My father clearly knows my situation in my school"). Reliability analysis showed that this scale was reliable (alpha=0.76). Identical items were used to assess maternal knowledge and formed the Maternal Knowledge Scale (alpha=0.79). The total score of the items in each scale was used as an indicator of the level of parental knowledge of the child's behavior, with a higher score indicating a higher level of knowledge (8).
2. *Paternal Expectation Scale (PEXP) and Maternal Expectation Scale (MEXP):* Seven items were developed to form the Paternal Expectation Scale (e.g., "My father requires me to have good behavior in school"). Reliability analysis showed that this scale was reliable (alpha=0.66). Identical items were used to assess maternal expectation and formed the Maternal Expectation Scale (alpha=0.64). The total score of the items in each scale was used as an indicator of the level of parental expectation of the child's behavior, with a higher score indicating a higher level of expectation and requirement (8).

3. *Paternal Monitoring Scale (PMON) and Maternal Monitoring Scale (MMON):* Seven items were developed to form the Paternal Monitoring Scale (e.g., "My father actively understands my situation in school). Reliability analysis showed that this scale was reliable (alpha=0.78). Identical items were used to assess maternal monitoring and formed the Maternal Monitoring Scale (alpha=0.76). The total score of the items in each scale was used as an indicator of the level of parental monitoring of the child's behavior, with a higher score indicating a higher level of monitoring (8).
4. *Paternal Discipline Scale (PDIS) and Maternal Discipline Scale (MDIS):* Five items were developed to form the Paternal Discipline Scale (e.g., "When I study hard, my father praises me"). Reliability analysis showed that this scale was reliable (alpha=0.63). Identical items were used to assess maternal discipline and formed the Maternal Discipline Scale (alpha=0.68). The total score of the items in each scale was used as an indicator of the level of reasonable parental discipline of the child's behavior, with a higher score indicating a higher level of reasonable parental discipline of the child (8).
5. *Paternal Parenting Style Scale and Maternal Parenting Style Scale:* To assess global parental control, the Paternal Parenting Style Scale and Maternal Parenting Scales (20) were used. There are two dimensions in these scales, including responsiveness and demandingness. In this study, the Responsiveness Scale (13 items) and Demandingness Scale (7 items) were reliable with reference to the fathers (PRES=0.76 and PDEM=0.74, respectively) and mothers (MRES=0.76 and MDEM=0.75, respectively). The total score of the items in each scale was used as an indicator of the level of parental responsiveness or demandingness, with a higher score indicating more positive parental attributes (8).
6. *Paternal Psychological Control Scale (PPSY) and Maternal Psychological Control Scale (MPSY):* Ten items were developed to form the Paternal Psychological Control Scale (e.g., "My father always wants to change my thoughts"). Reliability analysis showed that this scale was reliable (alpha=0.88). Identical items were used to assess maternal psychological control and formed the Maternal Psychological Control Scale (alpha=0.90). The total score of the items in each scale was used as an indicator of the level of parental psychological control, with a higher score indicating a higher level of control (8).

Assessment of Parent-Child Relational Qualities: Four aspects of parent-child relational qualities were assessed:

1. *Paternal Trust of Children Scale (PTRU) and Maternal Trust of Children Scale (MTRU):* Five items were developed to assess the respondents' perceptions of their fathers' trust about themselves and formed the Paternal Trust of Children Scale (PTRU). Reliability analysis showed that this scale was reliable (alpha=0.74). Identical items were used to assess children's perception of maternal trust about themselves and formed the Maternal Trust of Children Scale (alpha=0.73). The total score of the items in each scale was used as an indicator of the level of perceived trust that the parents had about their children, with a higher score indicating a higher level of trust (12).

2. *Children's Trust of Father Scale (TRUF) and Children's Trust of Mother Scale (TRUM):* Five items were developed to assess the respondents' trust about their fathers and formed the Children's Trust of Father Scale. Reliability analysis showed that this scale was reliable (alpha=0.67). Identical items were used to assess children's perceived trust of their mothers and formed the Children's Trust of Mother Scale (alpha=0.67). The total score of the items in each scale was used as an indicator of the level of the respondents' perceived trust about their parents, with a higher score indicating a higher level of trust (12).
3. *Readiness to Communicate with the Father Scale (RCF) and Readiness to Communicate with the Mother Scale (RCM):* Two items were developed to assess the respondents' readiness to communicate with the father and formed the Readiness to Communicate with the Father Scale. Reliability analysis showed that this scale was reliable (alpha=0.75). Identical items were used to assess children's readiness to share with their mothers and formed the Readiness to Communicate with the Mother Scale (alpha=0.75). The total score of the items in each scale was used as an indicator of the readiness of the children to communicate with their parents, with a higher score indicating a higher level of readiness (12).
4. *Satisfaction with Paternal Control Scale (SATF) and Satisfaction with Maternal Control Scale (SATM):* Four items were developed to form the Satisfaction with Paternal Control Scale (e.g., "I feel that how my father disciplines me is reasonable"). Reliability analysis showed that this scale was reliable (alpha=0.78). Identical items were used to assess the respondent's satisfaction with maternal control and formed the Satisfaction with Maternal Control Scale (alpha=0.78). The total score of the items in each scale was used as an indicator of the level of satisfaction of the child regarding parental control, with a higher score indicating a higher level of satisfaction (12).

OUR FINDINGS

Regarding the responses of the participants to the items in the Chinese Hopelessness Scale, frequency analyses showed that roughly one-fifth of the respondents responded in the negative direction on the items (see Table 1). In particular, 38.5% of the respondents were of the view that things just did not work out the way they wanted them to be.

Results showed that age was weakly related to adolescent hopelessness ($r=0.09$, $p<0.0001$). Regarding gender differences, analysis using t-test showed that adolescent boys scored higher on hopelessness than did adolescent girls ($M=24.32$, $SD=11.55$ for boys; $M=20.93$, $SD=9.95$ for girls ($t=8.29$, $p<0.0001$). With reference to parental education (ranging from no education to university education with 8 categories), Spearman correlation showed a negative relationship involved ($r=-0.12$, $p<0.0001$ and -0.12, $p<0.0001$ for paternal education and maternal education level, respectively).

Results showed that adolescent hopelessness was related to the marital status of the parents. Analysis using t-test showed that adolescent hopelessness was lower in the Intact Family Group (i.e., parents were engaged in a legal marriage; $M=25.08$, $SD=10.58$) than did the Non-Intact Family Group (i.e., parents were divorced, separated or having other forms of relationship; M=28.22, SD=11.21; t=2.88, p<0.01).

Finally, it was found that students experiencing economic disadvantage (M=24.43, SD=11.49) were more hopeless than did students not experiencing economic disadvantage (M=22.40, SD=10.85; t=3.01, p<0.01).

Table 1. Percentages of responses to the abridged version of the Chinese Hopelessness Scale

	Item	True[a]	False[a]
1.	I look forward to the future with hope and enthusiasm.	21.3	78.7
2.	I might as well give up because I can't make things better for myself.	19.3	80.7
3.	My future seems dark to me.	18.0	82.0
4.	I just don't get the breaks, and there is no reason to believe I will in the future.	20.9	79.1
5.	All I can see ahead of me is unpleasantness rather than pleasantness.	16.2	83.8
6.	I don't expect to get what I really want.	21.3	78.7
7.	They just don't work out the way I want them to be.	38.5	61.5
8.	I never get what I want so it's foolish to want anything.	20.0	80.0
9.	It is very unlikely that I will get any real satisfaction in the future.	23.7	76.3
10.	There's no use in really trying to get something I want because I probably won't get it.	27.2	72.8

[a] "True" percentage = sum of percentages of responses to "Strongly Agree", "Moderately Agree" and "Slightly Agree". "False" percentage = sum of percentages of responses to "Strongly Disagree", "Moderately Disagree" and "Slightly Disagree".

Pearson correlation coefficients on the relationships between different measures of parental control and adolescent hopelessness are presented in Table 2. As several correlation analyses were conducted, a multi-stage Bonferroni correction procedure (21) was used.

Two observations could be highlighted from the findings. First, as predicted, while higher levels of behavioral control based on different measures were negatively related to adolescent hopelessness, psychological control was positively related to adolescent hopelessness. Second, the relationships between the two domains did not differ for the paternal and maternal variables.

Similarly, correlation analyses were also carried out to examine the relationships between parent-child relational qualities and hopelessness (Table 2). As predicted, parent-child relational qualities were negatively related to hopelessness for the paternal and maternal variables and there were no major differences between the paternal variables and maternal variables.

To examine the relative contribution of different measures of behavioral control and psychological control to adolescent hopelessness, multiple regression analyses were performed for paternal control and maternal control variables. Results showed that maternal psychological control was the strongest predictor (Table 3).

Table 2. Relationship between parental control and parent-child relational qualities measures and hopelessness

Variables	HOPEL	Variables	HOPEL
PKNO	-0.27*	MKNO	-0.24*
PEXP	-0.06 [a]	MEXP	-0.03ns
PMON	-0.16*	MMON	-0.16*
PDIS	-0.01ns	MDIS	-0.02ns
PDEM	-0.17*	MDEM	-0.15*
PPSY	0.34*	MPSY	0.30*
PTRU	-0.35*	MTRU	-0.33*
TRUF	-0.28*	TRUM	-0.30*
RCF	-0.24*	RCM	-0.24*
SATF	-0.28*	SATM	-0.26*

Measures of parental control: PKNO: Paternal Knowledge Scale. PEXP: Paternal Expectation Scale. PMON: Paternal Monitoring Scale. PDIS: Paternal Discipline Scale. PDEM: Paternal Demandingness Scale. PPSY: Paternal Psychological Control Scale. MKNO: Maternal Knowledge Scale. MEXP: Maternal Expectation Scale. MMON: Maternal Monitoring Scale. MDIS: Maternal Discipline Scale. MDEM: Maternal Demandingness Scale. MPSY: Maternal Psychological Control Scale.

Measures of parent-child relational qualities: PTRU: Paternal Trust of Children Scale. TRUF: Children's Trust of Father Scale. RCF: Readiness to Communicate with Father Scale. SATF: Satisfaction with Paternal Control Scale. MTRU: Maternal Trust of Children Scale. TRUM: Children's Trust of Mother Scale. RCM: Readiness to Communicate with Mother Scale. SATM: Satisfaction with Maternal Control Scale.

A two-tailed multistage Bonferroni procedure was used to obtain the data related to all the correlations. pFW is based on the familywise Type 1 error rate. pT is the Type 1 error rate per test.

[*] pFW <0.01; pT<0.001. [a] Borderline significance; pT < .01.

Table 3. Predictors of hopelessness based on parental control measures

DV	Predictor Variables	Beta		R^2
Hopelessness	FKNO	-0.17	***	
	FEXP	0.01	ns	
	FMON	-0.04	ns	
	FDIS	-0.03	ns	
	FDEM	-0.05	*	
	FPSY	0.29	***	0.15
Hopelessness	MKNO	-0.15	***	
	MEXP	0.04	ns	
	MMON	-0.08	**	
	MDIS	-0.02	ns	
	MDEM	-0.05	*	
	MPSY	0.28	***	0.14

Note. PKNO: Paternal Knowledge Scale. PEXP: Paternal Expectation Scale. PMON: Paternal Monitoring Scale. PDIS: Paternal Discipline Scale. PDEM: Paternal Demandingness Scale. PPSY: Paternal Psychological Control Scale. MKNO: Maternal Knowledge Scale. MEXP: Maternal Expectation Scale. MMON: Maternal Monitoring Scale. MDIS: Maternal Discipline Scale. MDEM: Maternal Demandingness Scale. MPSY: Maternal Psychological Control Scale.

***p<0.0001. **p<0.001. *p<0.05.

ns-non-significant.

For the contribution of parent-child relational qualities to adolescent hopelessness, parental trust and trust of parents were the most important predictors (Table 4).

Table 4. Predictors of hopelessness based on parent-child relational qualities measures

DV	Predictor Variables	Beta	R^2
Hopelessness	PTRU	-0.24 ***	
	TRUF	-0.08 **	
	RCF	-0.06 **	
	SATF	-0.07	
			0.14
Hopelessness	MTRU	-0.27 ***	
	TRUM	-0.12 ***	
	RCM	-0.07 **	
	SATM	-0.05 ns	
			0.13

Note. PTRU: Paternal Trust of Children Scale. TRUF: Children's Trust of Father Scale. RCF: Readiness to Communicate with Father Scale. SATF: Satisfaction with Paternal Control Scale. MTRU: Maternal Trust of Children Scale. TRUM: Children's Trust of Mother Scale. RCM: Readiness to Communicate with Mother Scale. SATM: Satisfaction with Maternal Control Scale.
***$p<0.0001$.
**$p<0.001$.
ns -non-significant.

DISCUSSION

The purpose of this paper was to study the sense of hopelessness in Chinese adolescents in Shanghai and to identify the related socio-demographic correlates. There are several unique characteristics of the study. First, as there are few studies on adolescent hopelessness in China, the study is a pioneer attempt in the country. Second, the sample size is large and the related findings are based on students randomly sampled from schools in Shanghai. Third, validated Chinese measures were employed in the study. Finally, both socio-demographic and family variables were examined in the study. Based on the responses of the participants to the items in the abridged version of the Chinese Hopelessness Scale, it was observed that a significant proportion of the participants responded in the negative direction. The present findings are generally consistent with the previous studies that roughly one-fifth of Chinese adolescents in Hong Kong showed signs of hopelessness (22).

Concerning the demographic correlates of adolescent hopelessness, results showed that age was weakly related to hopelessness. This finding is consistent with the previous findings that age was positively related to psychological symptoms (8). This can be explained by the fact that stressors and challenges, particularly those related to the academic domain, are increasing as adolescents mature. Consistent with the previous findings that boys displayed higher levels of hopelessness symptoms (8), the present findings also showed that Chinese adolescent boys displayed a higher level of hopelessness than did Chinese adolescent girls. This finding is interesting because it is not consistent with the general findings in the literature that the mental health of women is relatively poorer than that of men. The present findings may possibly be explained by the fact that Chinese parents generally have very high expectations about their sons and the chance of getting into mainstream universities in China is extremely competitive. Actually, life challenges are immense even for university graduates in China.

The present findings provide useful pointers for the development of youth development programs. First, it is important to consider the question of how hopelessness in Chinese adolescents can be reduced. Unfortunately, literature review shows that there are very few adolescent prevention and positive youth development programs in different Chinese contexts (23). One notable exception is the Project P.A.T.H.S. (24-28) which can be used to promote adolescent well-being. It is exciting to note that the Project P.A.T.H.S. was implemented in Shanghai for three years (29). Definitely, the related experiences set the necessary ground work for wider implementation of the project in mainland China.

Consistent with the previous findings that parental education was negatively related to adolescent psychological symptoms (30), the present findings also showed that parental education was negatively related to adolescent hopelessness. The present findings suggest that adolescents whose parents with lower educational level had higher risk in terms of adolescent hopelessness. This can be explained in terms of the resources that parents in different socio-economic classes possess. It can be conjectured that parents with better education generally have more resources which would eventually create more opportunities for their children, hence creating hope for them. Another explanation is that parents with higher education have better parenting skills and parent-child relational qualities (30) which would eventually facilitate the learning of their children.

The present findings showed that marital status of the parents was related to adolescent hopelessness, with those in intact families displaying lower levels of adolescent hopelessness. The present findings may be explained by the possibility that family processes in non-intact families are dysfunctional which would eventually impair the psychological well-being of adolescents. There are research findings showing that the psychological well-being of adolescents coming from different families differed. Spruijt, DeGoede and Vandervalk (31) showed that compared with intact families, children of discordant nuclear families displayed more physical and mental problems. Halfon and Newacheck (32) reported that the prevalence of a disabling mental health condition was higher in single-parent families than intact families. Spruijt and de Goede (33) showed that amongst stable intact families, conflict intact families, single-parent families, and stepfamilies, adolescents from single-parent families performed worst in terms of physical health, suicidal ideation, mental health, relational well-being, and employment condition. The present findings basically replicated the previous findings.

Finally, consistent with literature, students experiencing economic disadvantage displayed a higher level of hopelessness than did students experiencing no economic disadvantage. For example, in a 3-year longitudinal study, Shek (34) showed that participants experiencing economic disadvantage generally had more negative perceptions of parenting quality and parent-child relational quality than did adolescents not experiencing economic disadvantage. Emotional well-being was also shown to be different in adolescents with and without economic disadvantage. In response to Orthner's (35) comment that studies in poverty "has not been accorded the level of research attention as families in middle class" (p.589), the present study is a constructive response.

Consistent with our expectation, results showed that although parental behavioral control was negatively related to hopelessness, psychological control was positively related to hopelessness. Actually, Shek (36) showed that relative to those conditions in which one or none of the adolescents' parents was perceived to display high parental psychological control at Time 1, adolescent hopelessness at Time 2 was greater when both parents were perceived to display high levels of parental psychological control at Time 1. The multiple regression analyses further showed that relative to behavioral control, psychological control is a stronger predictor of adolescent hopelessness. These findings are consistent with the Western literature that parental psychological control impairs the psychological well-being of adolescent children.

For the relationships between different measures of parent-child relational quality and adolescent hopelessness, the related measures were negatively related to adolescent hopelessness. These findings are consistent with those reported by Shek and Lee (8) based on Chinese adolescents in Hong Kong. For the multiple regression analyses, the findings underscore the importance of the role of mutual trust between parents and their adolescent children in adolescent hopelessness. The findings are pioneer because studies on the relationship between mutual trust in parents and their adolescent children are almost non-existent in the literature.

There are two limitations of the study. In the first place, there are two problems regarding the use of self-report measures in this study. First, relationships amongst the variables may be explained in terms of common method variance. Second, the sole reliance on adolescent report of parental control and parent-child relational qualities may give an incomplete view of the nature of family processes. The second limitation of the study is that only cross-sectional data were collected. Obviously, cross-sectional data cannot give a definitive picture on the causal relationships between family processes and adolescent hopelessness. Actually, there are findings showing bidirectional influences between perceived parenting qualities and adolescent hopelessness. Evidently, parents responded to their adolescent's manifestations of hopelessness with poor parenting may intensify the sense of hopelessness in their children.

ACKNOWLEDGMENTS

The preparation for this paper and the study were financially supported by the Wofoo Foundation. This chapter is based upon a paper published in the International Journal on Disability and Human Development (Han XY, Shek DTL. Socio-demographic and family correlates of hopelessness amongst adolescents in Shanghai, China. Int J Disabil Hum Dev 2012;11(2):113-9). Permission has been obtained from the publisher to publish this modified version of the paper in this book.

REFERENCES

[1] Shek DTL. The spirituality of Chinese people. In: Bond MH, editor. Oxford handbook of Chinese psychology. New York: Oxford University Press, 2010:343-66.

[2] Highfield MF, Cason C. Spiritual needs of patients: are they recognized? Cancer Nurs 1983;6:187-92.

[3] Thompson I. Mental health and spiritual care. Nurs Stand 2002;17:33-8.

[4] Anandarajah G, Hight E. Spirituality and medical practice: using the HOPE questions as a practical tool for spiritual assessment. Am Fam Physician 2001;63:81-8.

[5] Dyer JA, Kreitman N. Hopelessness, depression and suicide intent in parasuicide. Br J Psychiatr 1984;156:395-9.
[6] Milnes D, Owens D, Blenkiron P. Problems reported by self-harm patients: perception, hopelessness, and suicidal intent. J Psychosomatic Res 2002;53:819-22.
[7] Stoelb M, Chiriboga J. A process model for assessing adolescent risk for suicide. J Adolescence 1998;21:359-70.
[8] Shek DTL, Lee TY. Hopelessness in Chinese adolescents in Hong Kong: demographic and family correlates. Int J Adolesc Med Health 2005;17:279-90.
[9] Shek DTL. Perceived parental control processes, parent-child relational qualities, and psychological well-being in Chinese adolescents with and without economic disadvantage. J Genet Psychol 2005;166:171-88.
[10] Garber J, Flynn C. Predictors of depressive cognitions in young adolescents. Cogn Ther Res 2001;25:353-76.
[11] Tanaka E, Sakamoto S, Ono Y, Fujihara S, Kitamura T. Hopelessness in a community population: factorial structure and psychosocial correlates. J Soc Psychol 1998;138:581-90.
[12] Shek DTL. Parent-adolescent trust and parent-adolescent relationships in Chinese families in Hong Kong: implications for parent education and family therapy. Am J Fam Ther 2010;38:251-65.
[13] Shek DTL. Quality of life of Chinese people in a changing world. Soc Indic Res 2010;95:357-61.
[14] Shek DTL. Quality of life research: responses to emerging issues in a changing world. Soc Indic Res 2011;100:371-4.
[15] Shek DTL. Adolescent positive mental health and psychological symptoms: a longitudinal study in a Chinese context. Psychologia 1998;41:217-25.
[16] Ran MS, Xiang MZ, Li J, Huang J, Chen EYH, Chan CLW, et al. Correlates of lifetime suicide attempts among individuals with affective disorders in a Chinese rural community. Arch Suicide Res 2007;11:119-27.
[17] Stewart SM, Felice E, Claassen C, Kennard BD, Lee PWH, Emslie GJ. Adolescent suicide attempters in Hong Kong and the United States. Soc Sci Med 2006;63:296-306.
[18] Beck AT, Weissman A, Lester D, Trexler L. The measurement of pessimism: the Hopelessness Scale. J Consult Clin Psychol 1974;42:861-865.
[19] Shek DTL. Measurement of pessimism in Chinese adolescents: the Chinese Hopelessness Scale. Soc Behav Pers 1993;21:107-19.
[20] Shek DTL. Parenting characteristics and adolescent psychological well-being: a longitudinal study in a Chinese context. Genet Soc Gen Psychol Monogr 1999;125:27-44.
[21] Larzelere RE, Mulaik SA. Single-sample tests for many correlations. Psychol Bull 1977;84:557-69.
[22] Shek DTL. Mental health of secondary school students in Hong Kong: an epidemiological study using the General Health Questionnaire. Inter J Adolesc Med Health 1988;3:191-215.
[23] Shek DTL, Yu L. A review of validated youth prevention and positive youth development programmes in Asia. Int J Adolesc Med Health 2011;23:317-24.
[24] Shek DTL, Sun RCF. Effectiveness of the Tier 1 Program of Project P.A.T.H.S.: findings based on three years of program implementation. Sci World J 2010;10:1509-19.
[25] Shek DTL, Ma CMS. Impact of the Project P.A.T.H.S. in the junior secondary school years: individual growth curve analyses. Sci World J 2011;11:253-66.
[26] Shek DTL, Yu L. Prevention of adolescent problem behavior: longitudinal impact of the Project P.A.T.H.S. in Hong Kong. Sci World J 2011;11:546-67.
[27] Shek DTL, Ng CSM, Tsui PF. Qualitative evaluation of the Project P.A.T.H.S.: findings based on focus groups. Int J Disabil Hum Dev 2010;9:307-14.
[28] Shek DTL, Ng CSM. Early identification of adolescents with greater psychosocial needs: an evaluation of the Project P.A.T.H.S. in Hong Kong. Int J Disabil Hum Dev 2010;9:291-300.
[29] Shek DTL, Han XY, Ma HK. Positive Youth development curriculum (vols. 1-3). PATHS – Shanghai. Shanghai: Xue Lin Publishing Company, 2010.
[30] Shek DTL. Perceived parental control and parent-child relational qualities in Chinese adolescents in Hong Kong. Sex Roles 2005;53:635-46.

[31] Spruijt E, DeGoede M, Vandervalk I. The well-being of youngsters coming from six different family types. Patient Educ Counsel 2001;45:285-94.
[32] Halfon N, Newacheck PW. Prevalence and impact of parent-reported disabling mental health conditions among U.S. children. J Am Acad Child Adolesc Psychiatr 1999;38:600-9.
[33] Spruijt E, de Goede M. Transitions in family structure and adolescent well-being. Adolescence 1997;32:897-911.
[34] Shek DTL. Economic disadvantage, perceived family life quality, and emotional well-being in Chinese adolescents: a longitudinal study. Soc Indic Res 2008;85:169-89.
[35] Orthner DK. Families in poverty: key issues for research. J Fam Issues 1996;17:588-92.
[36] Shek DTL. A longitudinal study of perceived parental psychological control and psychological well-being in Chinese adolescents in Hong Kong. J Clin Psychol 2007;63:1-22.

In: Adolescence and Behavior Issues in a Chinese Context ISBN: 978-1-62618-614-9
Editors: DTL Shek, RCF Sun and Joav Merrick

Chapter 4

INTERNET ADDICTION IN HONG KONG ADOLESCENTS: PROFILES AND PSYCHOSOCIAL CORRELATES

***Daniel TL Shek**, PhD, FHKPS, BBS, JP*[1-5] *and Lu Yu, PhD*[1]**
[1]Department of Applied Social Sciences,
The Hong Kong Polytechnic University, Hong Kong, PRC
[2]Public Policy Research Institute, The Hong Kong Polytechnic University,
Hong Kong, PRC
[3]Deapartment of Social Work, East China Normal University, Shanghai, PRC
[4]Kiang Wu Nursing College of Macau, Macau, PRC
[5]Division of Adolescent Medicine, Department of Pediatrics,
Kentucky Children's Hospital, University of Kentucky College of Medicine,
Lexington, KY, US

ABSTRACT

This chapter examines the prevalence of Internet addition among Hong Kong adolescents and its psychosocial correlates in a large sample of early adolescents in Hong Kong. A total of 3,328 students (age = 12.59 ± 0.74 years) were recruited from 28 secondary schools in Hong Kong. Using Young's 10-item Internet Addiction Test, 26.4% of the participants were classified as having Internet addiction. Age and having divorced parents were positively correlated with pathological use of Internet, while higher academic competence, general positive youth development, and positive and clear identity predicted a lower probability of Internet addiction. These results demonstrate that Internet addiction has become an emergent youth problem in Hong Kong, which deserves more attention from researchers and professionals. Preventive strategies aiming at risk and protective factors identified in the present study should be developed and implemented.

* Correspondence: Professor Daniel T.L. Shek, PhD, FHKPS, BBS, JP, Chair Professor of Applied Social Sciences, Faculty of Health and Social Sciences, Department of Applied Social Sciences, The Hong Kong Polytechnic University, Room HJ407, Core H, Hung Hom, Hong Kong. E-mail: daniel.shek@polyu.edu.hk.

INTRODUCTION

The Internet has been described as one of the most important invention of the twentieth century. The use of Internet has dramatically changed the way people interact with others, gather and disseminate information, do business and entertainment. Meanwhile, a negative side of this new tool is emerging: addictive behaviors are fostered with the increasing use of Internet. Although there are different conceptions and definitions of Internet addiction, the term has been conceived as an individual's inability to control his or her use of the Internet (including any online-related, compulsive behavior) which eventually causes one's marked distress and functional impairment in daily life (1). Research findings have shown that excessive use of the Internet adversely affected one's physical health, family life and academic performance (2,3,4). In recent years, it has been reported that the risk of Internet addiction in adolescents continues to grow across the world (5). The present study was intended to provide a descriptive profile of Internet addictive behaviors among Hong Kong adolescents and to examine the psychosocial correlates of this phenomenon in a Chinese context.

A number of prevalence studies on Internet addiction have been conducted in different parts of the world where different findings were reported (6). In the United States, a national telephone survey showed that 5.9% of the respondents suffered from excessive Internet use, 3.7% felt preoccupied by the Internet when offline, 13.7% found it was difficult to stay away from the Internet for several days at a time, and 12.4% was found to stay online longer than intended very often or often (7). In the United Kingdom, a study based on 371 randomly selected students showed that 18.3% of the sample was diagnosed as problematic Internet users (8). With a sample of 3,237 adolescents from Norway, it was found that 1.98% and 8.68% could be regarded as having Internet addiction and at risk of Internet abuse, respectively (9).

Some important prevalence studies have been carried out in Asian countries, including different Chinese communities. Using an indigenous instrument, South Korean researchers found 4% and 20.4% of the adolescent respondents (N = 627) were high-risk Internet users and potential risk Internet users, respectively (10). Great concerns about Internet addiction are also shown in China because of the dramatic increase of Internet use among Chinese adolescents in the last decade. According to a national report in 2007, there were around 10 million Chinese teenagers who met the Internet addiction diagnostic criteria (11). A study on 2,620 high school students in Changsha showed that 2.4% of them could be diagnosed as Internet addicted (12). In another study where 3,557 first-year university students in Shanxi were recruited, 6.44% of the respondents were classified as Internet addictive users (13). In Taiwan, a study with a sample of 1,708 high school adolescents showed that 13.8% of the respondents were identified as Internet addicts, who were found to have different psychological and psychiatric problems (14).

With regard to Hong Kong, utilizing the Young's 20-item questionnaire to examine Internet addiction among 976 students, the Tsuen Wan Centre of the Chinese YMCA of Hong Kong (15) reported that 61.4% of senior primary school students, 35.2% of Secondary 1 to 3 students, 18.8% of Secondary 4 to 5 students, 35.8% of Secondary 6 to 7 students, and 37.0% of college students could be identified as highly at risk of Internet addiction. By comparing the data derived from two studies using the Young's 8-item questionnaire, Chan (16) found that the prevalence of Internet addiction had increased from 3.0% in 2000 to 14.7% in 2002. In a more recent study of 6,121 adolescents, Shek, Tang and Lo (17) showed that 19.1% of the respondents were Internet addicts using a validated Young's 10-item questionnaire.

While the number of prevalence studies on Internet addiction is accumulating, several conceptual and methodological gaps are observed. First, inconsistent findings regarding the prevalence rates of Internet addiction were reported by different researchers. Second, different instruments for assessing Internet addiction were used. For example, while a 40-item Chinese Internet-Related Addictive Behavior Inventory was designed and used to assess Internet addiction in Taiwan (14), Young's questionnaires were commonly adopted by researchers in China mainland and Hong Kong (13,18). Third, different diagnostic criteria and cut-off scores were employed in different studies. Although most studies followed Young's proposed cut-off of 4 of 10 symptoms criterion, some used a higher cut-off score. Fourth, most studies utilized cross-sectional designs and thus cannot provide a complete understanding of how Internet addiction developed. Fifth, some prevalence studies were based on small and unrepresentative samples. For example, in a study conducted in Korea aimed at analyzing causes of juvenile Internet addiction, only 240 completed questionnaires were collected out of 700 questionnaires distributed, which put both the reliability and validity of the findings in doubt (19). These gaps point to a critical need to establish standardized measures for the assessment of Internet addiction and to develop norms and cut-off scores for particular populations through methodologically sound empirical studies. Unfortunately, except a few exceptions (17), there are few validated Chinese measures on Internet addiction.

Against this background, the first purpose of the present study is to provide a descriptive profile of Internet addictive behavior among Hong Kong adolescents based on a large sample of Hong Kong students. The first wave of data of a large-scale longitudinal research (N = 3,328) in the continuation phase of the Project P.A.T.H.S. collected in the 2009-2010 academic year are presented in this paper. Obviously, such a descriptive profile would serve as a baseline profile for the next step longitudinal research. A validated instrument, Young's 10-item Internet addiction questionnaire, is used, which has shown robust psychometric properties on Hong Kong youth population in previous studies (17). It is expected that based on the longitudinal data, norms and cut-off scores for Internet addiction for Hong Kong adolescents would be eventually developed.

To prevent the intensified Internet addiction problem in adolescents, one important strategy is to reduce the related risk factors and strengthen the associated protective factors simultaneously. Hence, to devise effective preventive strategies, it is important first to understand both risk and protective factors in the development of Internet addiction. A few demographic factors were found to be related to Internet addiction. First, gender is correlated with the prevalence of Internet addiction. A common finding is that there are significantly more males than females who were identified as Internet addicts although the number of females involving in excessive Internet use also increased (20,21). Second, age has been consistently reported as a predictor of Internet addiction. Individuals who are in adolescence and young adulthood are more likely to become Internet addicts, as compared to other age groups (20,22). There are views suggesting that adolescents who are in the process of psychological development and crystallizing their personality may be particularly vulnerable to developing addictive behaviors. Researchers have also pointed out some other risk factors specific to this age group, including a strong desire to develop a sense of identity, a need to build up intimate relationship, and easily having access to the Internet either at home or in school (23). However, the relationship between age and Internet addiction within adolescence has not been addressed.

Third, parental marital discord is a risk factor for Internet addiction. It was reported that Internet addiction was more prevalent among adolescents who grew up in single-parent families, had high parent-adolescent conflict, and had inter-parental conflict (24). Fourth, with specific reference to Hong Kong, a society made up of immigrants, researchers have suggested that immigration status may be a risk factor for youth mental health (25). It has been reported that immigrant youth from mainland China often encountered acculturative stresses such as language difficulty and unfamiliarity with social resources, which may further lead to peer relationship problems and low self-image (26). As such, it is very likely that immigrant youth would display more behavioral problems than local youth, including Internet addiction. Nonetheless, the association between immigration status and adolescent Internet addictive behaviors remains to be investigated, especially in the context of Hong Kong.

Positive youth development may be another significant protective factor for adolescent Internet addiction. Researchers have reported that youth addictive behaviors such as gambling and substance abuse could be more effectively prevented by promoting positive youth development, such as pro-social behaviors, social competence, academic performance, and positive self-identity. For example, based on a two-year longitudinal dataset, Shek reported that positive youth development indexed by different indicators was negatively related to adolescent behavioral intention to gamble, and that positive youth development measures predicted adolescent gambling and their changes over time (27).

There are also cross-sectional as well as longitudinal findings showing that positive youth development indirectly influenced problem behavior via life satisfaction (28,29).

Similarly, researchers evaluated the long-term effects of an intervention that incorporate parental education, teacher training and social competence training on adolescent health risk behaviors for elementary school students living in high-crime communities (30). The results showed that students who received the intervention reported fewer delinquent behaviors by age 18. With regard to the prevention of Internet addiction, Shek and Yu recently reported the long-term effects of a positive youth development program, the Project P.A.T.H.S., on a list of youth problem behaviors, based on a longitudinal randomized group study (31).

The results showed that participants' ability to control Internet use in the control group decreased more quickly than the experimental group who received the positive youth development program and also showed a faster deceleration. Using the individual curve modeling technique, it was found that at the latter stage of the experiment while the program participants' control over Internet increased, such ability in the controlled participants continued to deteriorate. These findings suggest that positive youth development appear to be a common protective factor for youth problem behaviors, including Internet addiction. However, studies that directly examine the relationship between various positive youth development constructs and Internet addiction are almost non-existential.

Against this background, the second purpose of this study is to investigate risk and protective factors for Internet addiction in Hong Kong adolescents, with particular reference to gender, age, immigration status, parental marital status, and positive youth development.

Based on literature review, the following hypotheses are proposed: (1) male students would be more likely than female students to display Internet addictive behaviors; (2)

growing up in a non-intact family would be positively correlated with Internet addictive behavior; (3) immigrant youth would display more pathological Internet use than local adolescents; (4) different positive youth development constructs would be negatively related to adolescents' Internet misuse.

The identification of the relationship between these factors and the incidence of Internet addiction would be useful to develop effective approaches to prevent Internet addiction among adolescents in the future.

OUR STUDY

As introduced earlier, the present study is part of a large longitudinal study aiming at tracking the developmental trends of different positive youth development indicators and risk behaviors among Hong Kong adolescents over time. A total of 28 secondary schools in Hong Kong were selected to participate in the study. Data regarding Internet addiction behaviors collected in the first wave of this study are analyzed in this paper.

Participants

All Secondary 1 students in the selected schools were invited to complete a questionnaire anonymously. There were 3,328 students responding to the questionnaire. The mean age of the participants was 12.59 years (SD = 0.74). These included 1,719 boys, 1,572 girls, and 37 students who did not indicate their gender. While most students were born in Hong Kong (78.3%), there were 19.8% of the participants from China Mainland and 1.9% from other places. The background demographic information of the participants is summarized in Table 1.

Procedures

In the school year of 2009-2010, the participants were invited to respond to a comprehensive youth development questionnaire including both existing instruments and scales developed by the first author. The questionnaire survey was conducted by a trained research assistant in classroom settings with standardized instructions.

At each measurement occasion, the purposes of the study were introduced and confidentiality of the data collected was repeatedly ensured to all participants. School, parental and student consent had been obtained before data collection. Participants responded to the questionnaires in a self-administered format. The research assistant was present throughout the administration process to answer possible questions from the participants.

Table 1. Descriptive statistics about participants

Categorical variables	n	%	
Gender			
Male	1,719	52.2%	
Female	1,572	47.8%	
Place of birth			
Hong Kong	2,590	78.3%	
Mainland China	655	19.8%	
Others	64	1.9%	
Parental marital status			
First marriage	2781	84.4%	
Divorced	209	6.3%	
Separated	73	2.2%	
Remarried	129	3.9%	
Others (not first marriage)	104	3.2%	
Family economic status			
Receiving CSSA	225	6.8%	
Not receiving CSSA	2606	78.3%	
Others	465	13.9%	
Internet addiction			
Yes	847	26.4%	
No	2364	73.6%	
Continuous variables	Mean	SD	Range
Age	12.59	0.74	10-18
ASC	3.12	0.67	1-5
CBC	4.45	0.75	1-6
PA	4.50	0.89	1-6
GPYDQ	4.50	0.71	1-6
PIT	4.24	0.96	1-6
NET	0.23	0.24	0-1

Notes: CSSA = Comprehensive Social Security Assistance.
ASC = academic school competence; CBC = cognitive behavioral competence;
PA = prosocial attributes; GPYDQ = general positive youth development qualities;
PIT = positive identity; NET = Internet addiction.

Instruments

Participants were invited to respond to a composite questionnaire that comprises questions about demographic information, participants' family environment, different measures of youth development constructs and problem behaviors.

For family factors, participants responded to questions regarding paternal presence, maternal presence, parental marital status, paternal educational level, maternal educational level, and family economic status. Family economic status is indexed by the question of whether the family of the participant is receiving Comprehensive Social Security Assistance (CSSA), a financial aid provided by Hong Kong Government for low-income populations, at the time of survey. Respondents were also asked to indicate the marital status of their parents, including: "divorced and not remarried", "separate and not remarried", "couple, first marriage", "couple, second or above marriage", and "others".

The scales used to assess Internet addiction and positive youth development constructs are introduced below. Internal consistency of each measure for the present sample is summarized in Table 4.

Young's 10-item Internet Addiction Test (IAT)

Young developed several instruments to assess Internet addiction, among which the 10-item Internet Addiction Test has been validated by Shek, Tang and Chan (17) for Chinese populations and was selected to measure youth Internet addictive behavior in this study. The 10-item IAT asks respondents to answer "Yes" or "No" as to whether they have the listed Internet addictive behaviors in the past one year. Example items include "feeling a need to spend more and more time online to achieve satisfaction" and "feeling restless or irritable when attempting to cut down or stop on-line use". A person is classified as "Internet addiction" if he/she shows 4 or more of the listed behaviors. Cronbach's alpha of IAT for the present sample was 0.79.

Chinese Positive Youth Development Scale (CPYDS)

The CPYDS consists of 15 subscales which are listed as follows:

1. Bonding Subscale (three items)
2. Resilience Subscale (three items)
3. Social Competence Subscale (three items)
4. Emotional Competence Subscale (three items)
5. Cognitive Competence Subscale (three items)
6. Behavioral Competence Subscale (three items)
7. Moral Competence Subscale (three items)
8. Self-Determination Subscale (three items)
9. Self-Efficacy Subscale (two items)
10. Beliefs in the Future Subscale (three items)
11. Clear and Positive Identity Subscale (three items)
12. Spirituality Subscale (three items)
13. Prosocial Involvement Subscale (three items)
14. Prosocial Norms Subscale (three items)
15. Recognition for Positive Behavior Subscale (three items)

Based on factor analyses, Shek and Ma (32) proposed that the 15 subscales in the CPYDS could be further reduced to four dimensions:

- Cognitive Behavioral Competence (CBC): Scale score is calculated by averaging scores on Cognitive Competence Subscale, Self-Determination Subscale, and Behavioral Competence Subscale.
- Prosocial Attributes (PA): Scale score equals to the mean score of Prosocial Involvement Subscale and Prosocial Norms Subscale.
- Positive Identity (PIT): Scale score is computed by averaging scores of Beliefs in the Future Subscale and Clear and Positive Identity Subscale.
- General Positive Youth Development Qualities (GPYDQ): Scale score equals to the mean score of Resilience Subscale, Social Competence Subscale, Self-Efficacy Subscale, Moral Competence Subscale, Bonding Subscale, Recognition for Positive Behavior Subscale, Spirituality Subscale, and Emotional Competence Subscale.

These four composite indicators were used to assess participants' positive youth development in the present study. Scores of the four indicators all range from 1 to 6 with higher scores representing for high competences in the constructs. Descriptive statistics about all variables under study are listed in Table 1. It should be noted that although the administered questionnaire includes other subscales of the CPYDS, findings regarding the overall score of CPYDS and its subscales will be reported elsewhere. The present paper only focused on the predictive effects of the four second-order positive youth development constructs on adolescent Internet addictive behaviors.

Academic and school competence scale

As a relatively independent positive youth development construct, participants' academic and school competence (ASC) were measured by three items. For the first item, participants are required to rate their perceived academic performance as compared to other peer students on a five-point Likert scale, with "1" = "very poor", "2" = "below average", "3" = "average", "4" = "above average", and "5" = "very good". The second item asks the extent to which the respondents are satisfied with their academic performance ("1" = "very dissatisfied", "2" = "dissatisfied", "3" = "neutral", "4" = "satisfied", and "5" = "very satisfied").

The last question asks the participants to rate their conduct in school on a five-point Likert scale ("1" = "very poor", "2" = "below average", "3" = "average", "4" = "above average", and "5" = "very good"). The ASC scale score is calculated by averaging the item scores and ranges from 1 to 5, with high scores representing for high academic and school competence.

Data analytic plan

The first purpose of the present study was to provide a descriptive profile of different Internet additive behaviors among Hong Kong adolescents. Therefore, numbers and percentages of adolescents who reported pathological use of Internet were first computed. Second, to investigate whether gender, age, immigration status, and positive youth development are predictive of adolescent Internet addictive behaviors, multiple regression analysis was performed with the mean score of IAT items as the dependent variable.

Specifically, basic demographic factors (age and gender) were entered in the first block; family economic status, parental marital status, and immigration status of the participant were entered into the second block; youth development constructs including academic and school competence (ASC), cognitive behavioral competence (CBC), prosocial attributes (PA), positive identity (PIT), and general positive youth development qualities (GPYDQ) were entered into the third block of the regression model.

To further determine whether different demographic factors and positive youth development constructs contribute to the occurrence of Internet addiction, a logistic regression analysis was conducted. Participants who met Young's criterion of Internet addiction were first identified. Whether the participant can be diagnosed as Internet addiction served as the dependent variable. Independent variables and the order of input were the same as those in the multiple regression analysis.

It should be noted that although the relationship between family economic status and Internet addiction was not a major focus of the present study, this variable was also included as an independent predictor throughout the analyses to control for its possible effects.

As 465 participants did not indicate whether their family was receiving CSSA in the year of survey, they were not included in the correlation analyses. In addition, because immigrant youth from other places than mainland China only accounted for 1.9% of the participants, they were also not included in the analyses that investigated the relationship between immigration status and Internet addiction. In other words, the present study focused on comparing local and immigrant adolescents from mainland China.

OUR FINDINGS

In this part, descriptive profile of different type of Internet addictive behavior is presented first, followed by the results of multiple regression analyses regarding the predictive effects of demographic characteristics, immigration status, and positive youth development constructs of the participated students on their Internet addictive behaviors.

Finally, relationships between different predictors and the occurrence of Internet addiction at the diagnostic level are reported.

Descriptive profiles on Internet addictive behavior

Numbers and percentages of participants who displayed Internet addictive behaviors in the past one year are summarized in Table 2. Several observations can be highlighted from the findings. First, Internet addictive behaviors are quite common among Hong Kong adolescents. For example, 39.9% of the respondents reported "feeling preoccupied with the Internet or online services and think about it while off-line"; 42.4% of the students "stay online longer than originally intended"; and about 19.5% of the participants "risk the loss of a significant relationship, job, or educational or career opportunity because of online use". Second, according to Young's criterion, 26.4% of the respondents can be classified as Internet addiction. Third, 19.2% of the students reported to "go online to escape problems or relieve feelings such as helplessness, guilt, anxiety or depression", which indicates the possible psychological and psychiatric comorbidity. These figures clearly highlight the fact that Internet addiction is a growing problem for Hong Kong adolescents.

Correlates of Internet addictive behavior

First, to provide a general picture of the relationships among different variables, several basic statistical analyses were performed. Means and standard deviations for the variables under study are shown in Table 1. For the dependent variable, i.e., Internet Addiction Test (IAT) scale score, descriptive statistics by different groups of gender, family economic status, parental marital status, and immigration status are summarized in Table 3. Pearson correlation coefficients among positively youth development constructs and Internet addiction are also calculated and presented in Table 4. Second, the predictive effects of participants' demographic variables and positive youth development constructs on pathological use of Internet were examined in a multiple regression model.

Table 2. Percentage of participants with Internet addictive behavior

Internet use behaviors in the past year	No		Yes	
	Number	Percent	Number	Percent
1. Feeling preoccupied with the Internet or on-line services and think about it while off-line	1,993	60.1%	1,324	39.9%
2. Feeling a need to spend more and more time on-line to achieve satisfaction	2,243	67.7%	1,072	32.3%
3. Unable to control your on-line use	2,561	77.3%	752	22.7%
4. Feeling restless or irritable when attempting to cut down or stop on-line use	2,824	85.4%	484	14.6%
5. Stay on-line longer than originally intended?	1,906	57.6%	1,404	42.4%
6. Risk the loss of a significant relationship, job, or educational or career opportunity because of on-line use	2,659	80.5%	644	19.5%
7. Lie to family members or friends to conceal excessive Internet use	2,658	80.3%	651	19.7%
8. Go on-line to escape problems or relieve feelings such as helplessness, guilt, anxiety or depression	2,666	80.8%	633	19.2%
9. Showing withdrawal when off-line, such as increased depression, moodiness, or irritability	2,902	88.0%	395	12.0%
10. Keep on using Internet even after spending too much money on on-line fees	2,962	89.9%	331	10.1%
Participants can be classified as Internet addiction (Young's criteria)	**2,364**	**73.6%**	**847**	**26.4%**

Table 3. Means and standard deviations of Internet addiction in different groups by gender, immigrant status, family economic status and parental marital status

	Internet addiction	
	Mean	Standard Deviation
Overall	0.23	0.24
Gender		
Male	0.24	0.25
Female	0.22	0.23
Immigrant status		
Hong Kong	0.22	0.23
Mainland China	0.26	0.25
Family economic status		
Not receiving CSSA	0.23	0.24
Receiving CSSA	0.25	0.23
Parental marital status		
Divorced	0.28	0.26
Separated	0.25	0.22
Married	0.22	0.23
Remarried	0.26	0.24
Others	0.27	0.24

Note: Means and standard deviations in the table are based on scale scores of Internet Addiction Test.

Table 4. Correlations among variables and reliabilities of scales

	ASC	CBC	PA	GPYDQ	PIT	Cronbach's α (mean)[#]
ASC	--	--	--	--	--	.67 (.40)
CBC	.26	--	--	--	--	.82 (.61)
PA	.28	.60	--	--	--	.74 (.59)
GPYDQ	.37	.79	.74	--	--	.88 (.48)
PIT	.40	.71	.63	.75	--	.82 (.69)
NET	-.22	-.24	-.26	-.33	-.27	.79 (.28)

Note: NET: Internet addiction; ASC: academic and school competence; CBC: cognitive behavioral competence; PA: prosocial attributes; GPYDQ: general positive youth development qualities; PIT: positive identity.

All correlations are significant at the 0.01 level.

[#] Mean inter-item correlations.

The results are presented in Table 5. Several significant findings can be highlighted. First, participants' age was predictive of Internet addictive behaviors: older students tended to display more pathological use of Internet than younger students. Second, participants with divorced parents were more likely to show Internet addictive behaviors than participants with intact family. Third, higher academic and school adjustment, general positive youth development score, and positive and clear identity significantly predicted a lower level of pathological use of Internet.

Table 5. Multiple regression analyses on students' Internet addictive behavior

	B	Beta	Sig	R^2	R^2 change
First block					
Age	**0.02**	**0.05**	**.01**		
Gender	-0.01	-0.02	.40	.01	.01*
Second block					
Immigration status	0.02	0.04	.10		
Family economic status	0.00	0.00	.96		
Parental marital status					
Parent_divorced	**0.05**	**0.05**	**.02**		
Parent_separated	-0.01	-0.01	.71		
Parent_remarried	0.04	0.03	.15		
Parent_others	-0.02	-0.01	.52	.01	.01*
Third block					
ASC	**-0.04**	**-0.11**	**.00**		
CBC	0.01	0.04	.23		
PA	-0.01	-0.03	.28		
GPYDQ	**-0.09**	**-0.27**	**.00**		
PIT	**-0.01**	**-0.07**	**.04**	.15	.13**

Notes: * $p < .01$ ** $p < .001$

Immigration status: 1 = immigrant from mainland China; 0 = local participant.

Family economic status: 1 = Receiving Comprehensive Social Security Assistance (CSSA); 2 = not receiving CSSA.

ASC = academic school competence; CBC = cognitive behavioral competence; PA = prosocial attributes; GPYDQ = general positive youth development qualities; PIT = positiveidentity.

Fourth, unexpectedly, both gender and immigration status did not show significant relationship with participants' Internet addiction. Fifth, the effect of family economic status on Internet misuse was non-significant. The whole model explained 15% of the variance in adolescents' Internet addictive behaviors.

Predictors of the occurrence of Internet addiction

The results of logistic regression analysis are presented in Table 6. Using the probability of being diagnosed as Internet addiction as the dependent variable, three factors are found to be significant predictors. First, having divorced parents increased the probability of meeting the diagnostic criterion of Internet addiction, with an odds ratio of 1.77 ($p = 0.01$).

This indicates that students with divorced parents were 1.77 times more likely to be diagnosed as Internet addiction than students whose parents were in their first marriage. The second factor is academic and school competence. Participants who scored higher on academic performance were less likely to be classified as Internet addiction (OR = 0.69, $p < .001$). Third, general positive youth development qualities score served as a protective factor for Internet addiction, with an odds ratio of 0.46 ($p < .001$). This means that when the participant's score on general positive youth development constructs increases one point, the possibility of being diagnosed as Internet addiction would be reduced by half. Again, gender and immigration status were not significant predictors of Internet addiction.

Table 6. Logistic regression analyses on students' Internet addiction

	B	Odds Ratio	*p*
First block			
Age	0.05	1.05	.53
Gender	-0.08	0.93	.93
Second block			
Immigration status	0.16	1.17	.27
Family economic status (CSSA)	0.11	1.12	.59
Parental marital status			
Parent_divorced	**.57**	**1.77**	**.01**
Parent_separated	.14	1.15	.69
Parent_remarried	.40	1.50	.11
Parent_others	-.15	0.86	.64
Third block			
ASC	**-0.38**	**0.69**	**.00**
CBC	0.00	1.00	.99
PA	-0.05	0.95	.60
GPYDQ	**-0.79**	**0.46**	**.00**
PIT	-0.02	0.98	.80

Notes: Immigration status: 1 = immigrant from mainland China; 0 = local participant.

Family economic status: 1 = Receiving Comprehensive Social Security Assistance (CSSA); 2 = not receiving CSSA.

ASC = academic school competence; CBC = cognitive behavioral competence; PA = prosocial attributes; GPYDQ = general positive youth development qualities; PIT = positive identity.

Males and females showed similar probability of having Internet addiction; and the number of Internet addicts identified in immigrant adolescents from mainland China did not differ from that of local youth. These findings are basically consistent with the results of linear regression analysis.

DISCUSSION

This study suggests that Internet addictive behaviors in Hong Kong adolescent are prevalent. The results demonstrate that Internet addiction has become a serious youth development issue, which requires wider attention from helping professionals and policy makers. It was found that an older age was a risk factor for Internet addiction, while good academic and school performance, high general positive youth development qualities score, and positive self-identity predicted low level of Internet addictive behaviors. The identification of these factors would be helpful to develop preventive strategies for Internet addiction among local adolescents in Hong Kong. In particular, the use of positive youth development program can be regarded as a promising strategy in preventing Internet addiction.

Using Young's criterion, the present study found that 26.4% of the participated students can be identified as Internet addicts. The percentages of adolescents displaying different problematic Internet use behaviors ranged from 10.1% to 42.4%. Compared with previous prevalence data on Hong Kong adolescents, the present results are generally higher than the rates reported earlier by other researchers (16,17). Echoing Chan's study (16), this finding indicates that overuse of the Internet has become a serious problem for adolescent population in Hong Kong, and that the problem is intensified in recent years. Clearly, the increasing use of Internet in different areas for various purposes, easy accessibility of the Internet and implicit or explicit encouragement for Internet use for adolescents may contribute to the growing number of young Internet addicts. As with other addictive disorders, Internet addiction are associated with impaired peer and family relationship, low academic performance and a range of psychological problems, including depression, low self-esteem, high sense of loneliness, and compulsivity. Therefore, there is an urgent need in Hong Kong society for researchers, educators, parents and policy makers to work together to solve this issue.

Meanwhile, the Chinese version of Young's 10-item questionnaire demonstrated satisfying reliability and validity in the present study, as reflected in the high internal consistency and the negative relationships with a list of positive youth development constructs (i.e., evidence of construct validity). Different measures and cut-off criteria of Internet addiction have led to the inconsistent prevalence rates reported in the literature. Given the results of the present study, the validated Chinese version of Young's 10-item Internet addiction questionnaire appears to be a promising instrument to assess pathological use of Internet for Chinese people. Future studies may utilize a wider range of respondents from different Chinese populations to further establish norms and validate cut-off points for the interpretation of this scale based on rigorous research design. In addition, there is a need to look at the relationship between Internet addictive behavior and other clinical problems.

The present results also showed that with age increases, adolescents tend to display more Internet addictive behaviors. Previous studies suggest that compared to other age groups, Internet addiction is more likely to happen in adolescence and young adulthood because young people who are in the process of psychological and personality development may be particularly vulnerable to fostering addictive behaviors. It is possible that within adolescence, the desire to develop a sense of identity and the need to build up intimate relationship become increasingly stronger as adolesecents grow older (33). This may explain the finding that older adolescents showed more overuse of Internet than younger adolescents. In addition, older adolescents tend to have more accesses to the Internet either at home or in school than younger adolescents, which may also contribute to the positive association between age and Internet addictive behaviors. The findings also suggest that early identification and prevention are important.

An unpredicted finding of this study is that Internet addiction was unrelated to gender. Previous reports generally show that as with other addictive behaviors Internet addiction is more common in males than in females. For example, Chou and Hsiao reported that only three out of a total of 54 Internet addiction cases were female students based on a sample of more than 900 Taiwan college students (34). Scherer (35) found that dependent Internet users included a significant larger proportion of men (71%) to women (29%) than the non-dependent users (50% are men and women). As discussed earlier, different instruments and cut-off criteria of Internet addiction used in different studies may contribute to the inconsistent findings. In fact, researchers have reported that males and females used the Internet differently. For example, Young reported that men tended to seek out dominant activities online while women sought out close friendships and virtual communications online (36). Therefore, if the instrument mainly assesses the applications that are more frequently engaged by males, apparently there would be more males than females being diagnosed as

Internet addiction. Besides, there are views suggesting that gender difference in Internet addiction may simply due to the fact that more men than women use the Internet worldwide (21). This may not be the case in Hong Kong. According to a recent report (37), the percentage of male Internet users (51.9%) is only slightly higher than female users (48.1%) in Hong Kong. With reference to adolescent population, the difference may be even smaller. Thus, the existence of gender difference among adolescents with Internet addiction remains unclear and further work is needed.

It was found that having divorced parents significantly predicted Internet addictive behavior. This is consistent with our prediction that non-intact family status may be a risk factor for Internet addiction. Researchers have reported that children living with divorced parents tend to have high parent-adolescent conflicts and low levels of parent-child involvement, which would result in inadequate parental monitoring, and low family cohesion, which in turn would predict adolescents' Internet addictive behavior (38). Moreover, adolescents who have conflicts with their parents often refuse to conform to the supervision of parents, including rules set for Internet use. Lacking of support from parents, adolescents living with divorced parents may seek social support from the interacting experiences on the Internet. In fact, their excessive use of Internet may further aggregate their conflict with parents, which forms a vicious circle between poor parent-child relationship and Internet addiction, and makes the problem of addicting to Internet more difficult to solve (24). The observation is also consistent with the previous findings that parent-child relationship and psychological well-being in adolescents growing up in non-intact families were worse than those for adolescents in intact families (39,40).

Contrary to the hypothesis, immigrant youth from mainland China did not show more Internet addictive behaviors than local adolescents. This indicates that immigrant youth may not have worse mental health status than local students in Hong Kong, despite the difficulties they might have encountered during adaptation. Researchers have found that positive youth development constructs, such as social competence and resilience, would help adolescents to cope with stress and adversity in a positive manner and prevent them from mental health problems (41,42,43). It is possible that immigrant youth had a higher level of positive youth development than local students. In fact, this possibility has been supported by a recent study which showed that as compared to local youth, immigrant adolescents exhibited higher levels of self-control, empathy, assertiveness, and the ability to read social cues (44). It would be interesting to further compare other positive youth development indicators between local and immigrant adolescents, and to examine how these factors may contribute to the mental health of immigrant and local students respectively. While the present findings are intriguing, they must be interpreted with caution because students' immigration status in this study was measured by asking for their place of birth. Therefore, the identified immigrant youth actually include both new immigrants and those who have lived in Hong Kong for many years. These "old" immigrant adolescents may have been adapted to the Hong Kong society as well as local youth. Future research could focus on the mental health of new immigrant adolescents.

One of the most remarkable findings of the present study is the negative relationships between different positive youth development constructs and adolescent Internet addiction. Participants who had higher academic and school competence, and scored higher on general positive youth development qualities indicator and positive identity displayed less Internet addictive behaviors. This provides evidence for positive youth development as a protective factor for adolescent problem behavior, including Internet addiction. The implication is that

Internet addiction may be prevented through promoting positive youth development. Shek and Yu have reported that participants of the Project P.A.T.H.S., a program that aims to promote holistic positive development among adolescents, displayed higher levels of positive youth development and stronger ability to control Internet use, comparing to students without joining the program (30). However, the question of whether the improved self-control over Internet results from the enhancement of different positive youth development constructs is not directly examined. The present finding that positive youth development constructs significantly predicted low probability of Internet addiction provides a positive answer to this question. More in-depth studies are needed to further examine how positive youth development constructs help to prevent Internet addictive behaviors.

In summary, based on a large sample of secondary school students, this study examined the prevalence of Internet addiction among Hong Kong adolescents and its relationship with a variety of psychosocial factors. It demonstrated that problematic use of Internet has become an emergent youth problem in Hong Kong, which deserves more attention from researchers and professionals. It was found that age and having divorced parents were risk factors for youth Internet addiction and high academic competence, general positive youth development qualities, and positive identity prevented adolescents from developing Internet addiction. Preventive strategies must be developed and implemented in a timely manner, with the identified risk and protective factors being considered. Such prevention programs/policies could incorporate age-specific components. More importantly, programs that promote positive youth development, such as the Project P.A.T.H.S., may represent a promising direction for preventing Internet addiction among adolescents in the future (45,46). In view of the lack of preventive and positive youth development programs in Hong Kong (47,48,49), there is a need to re-think about how positive youth development may help to reduce adolescent developmental problems in Chinese adolescents.

ACKNOWLEDGMENTS

The preparation for this paper and the Project P.A.T.H.S. were financially supported by The Hong Kong Jockey Club Charities Trust. This chapter is based upon a paper published in the International Journal on Disability and Human Development (Shek DTL, Yu L. Internet addiction in Hong Kong adolescents: Profiles and psychosocial correlates. Int J Disabil Hum Dev 2012;11(2):133-42). Permission has been obtained from the publisher to publish this modified version of the paper in this book.

REFERENCES

[1] Young KS. Internet addiction: symptoms, evaluation, and treatment. In L. Van de Creek L, Jackson T, editors. Innovations in clinical practice: a source book, vol. 17. Sarasota, FL: Professional Resource Press, 1999:19-31.

[2] Young KS, Rogers RC. The relationship between depression and Internet addiction. Cyberpsychol Behav 1998; 1:25-28.

[3] Kaltiala-Heino R, Lintonen T, Rimpelä A. Internet addiction? Potentially problematic use of the Internet in a population of 12-18 year old adolescents. Addict Res Theory 2004;12: 89-96.

[4] Yen JY, Ko CH, Yen CF, Wu HY, Yang MJ. The comorbid psychiatric symptoms of Internet addiction: attention deficit and hyperactivity disorder (ADHD), depression, social phobia, and hostility. J Adolesc Health 2007;41(1):93-98.
[5] Young KS, Nabuco de Abreu C, editors. Internet addiction: a handbook and guide to evaluation and treatment. Hoboken, NJ: John Wiley & Sons, Inc, 2010.
[6] Beard KW. Internet addiction: a review of current assessment techniques and potential assessment questions. Cyberpsychol Behav 2005;8:7-14.
[7] Aboujaoude E, Koran LM, Gamel N, Large MD, Serpe RT. Potential markers for problematic Internet use: a telephone survey of 2,513 adults. CNS Spectr 2006;11:750-55.
[8] Niemz K, Griffiths M. Prevalence of pathological Internet use among University students and correlations with self-esteem, the General Health Questionnaire (GHQ), and disinhibition. Cyberpsychol Behav 2005;8:562-70.
[9] Johansson A, Götestam KG. Internet addiction: characteristics of a questionnaire and prevalence in Norwegian youth (12-18 years). Scand J Psychol 2004;45(3):223-29.
[10] Lee M, Ko Y, Song H, Kwon K, Lee H, Nam M, Jung I. Characteristics of Internet use in relation to game genre in Korean adolescents. Cyberpsychol Behav 2007;10:278-85.
[11] China Internet Network Information Center. Statistical Report on Internet Development in China 2009. China Internet Network Information Center, 2009. Retrieved from: http://www.cnnic.cn/
[12] Cao F, Su L. Internet addiction among Chinese adolescents: prevalence and psychological features. Child Care Health Dev 2007;33:275-81.
[13] Ni X, Yan H, Chen S, Liu Z. Factors influencing internet addiction in a sample of freshmen university students in China. Cyberpsychol Behav 2009;12:327-30.
[14] Yang SC, Tung CJ. Comparison of Internet addicts and non-addicts in Taiwanese high school. Comput Hum Behav 2007;23:79-96.
[15] Tsuen Wan Centre, Chinese YMCA of Hong Kong. Study on adolescents' Internet using behaviors. Hong Kong: Tsuen Wan Centre, Chinese YMCA of Hong Kong, 2004.
[16] Chan TCF. Cyber risk of Hong Kong youngsters. J Youth Stud 2004;7:155-68.
[17] Shek DTL, Tang VMY, Lo CY. Internet addiction in Chinese adolescents in Hong Kong: assessment, profiles, and psychosocial correlates. ScientificWorldJournal 2008;8:776-87.
[18] Leung L. Net-generation attributes and seductive properties of the Internet as predictors of online activities and Internet addiction. Cyberpsychol Behav 2004;7:333-48.
[19] Hur MH. Demographic, habitual, and socioeconomic determinants of Internet Addiction Disorder: an empirical study of Korean teenagers. Cyberpsychol Behav 2006;9:514-25.
[20] Griffiths MD. Internet addiction: Does it really exist? In Gackenbach J, editor. Psychology and the Internet: intrapersonal, interpersonal, and transpersonal implications. New York: Academic Press, 1998:61-75.
[21] Morahan-Martin JM, Schumacker P. Incidence and correlates of pathological Internet use. Comput Human Behav 2000;16:13-29.
[22] Kandell JJ. Internet addiction on campus: the vulnerability of college students. Cyberpsychol Behav 1998;1:11-17.
[23] Ary DV, Duncan TE, Biglan A, Metzler CW, Noell JW, Smolkowski K. Development of adolescent problem behavior. J Abnorm Child Psych 1999;27:141-50.
[24] Yen JY, Yen CF, Chen CC, Chen SH, Ko CH. Family factors of Internet addiction and substance use experience in Taiwanese adolescents. Cyberpsychol Behav 2007;10:323-329.
[25] The Hong Kong Federation of Youth Groups. The population poser: how do young new arrivals from mainland China adapt? Hong Kong: The Hong Kong Federation of Youth Groups, 1995.
[26] Chan J, editor. A survey study on the psychological adaptation of newly arrived students from mainland China. Hong Kong: Aberdeen Kai-Fong Welfare Association Social Service Centre, 1999.
[27] Shek DTL. Positive youth development and behavioral intention to gamble among Chinese adolescents in Hong Kong. Int J Adolesc Med Health 2010;22(1):163-72.
[28] Sun RCF, Shek DTL. Life satisfaction, positive youth development and problem behaviour among Chinese adolescents in Hong Kong. Soc Indic Res 2010;95(3):455-74.

[29] Sun RCF, Shek DTL. Positive youth development, life satisfaction and problem behavior among Chinese adolescents in Hong Kong: a replication. Soc Indic Res 2012;105:541-59.
[30] Hawkins JW, Brown EC, Oesterle S, Arthur MW, Abbott RD, Catalano RF. Early effects of Communities That Care on targeted risks and initiation of delinquent behavior and substance use. J Adolesc Health 2008;43:15-22.
[31] Shek DTL, Yu L. Prevention of adolescent problem behavior: longitudinal impact of the Project P.A.T.H.S. in Hong Kong. ScientificWorldJournal 2011;11:546-67.
[32] Shek DTL, Ma CMS. Dimensionality of the Chinese Positive Youth Development Scale: confirmatory factor analyses. Soc Indic Res 2010;98:41-59.
[33] Waterman AS. Identity development from adolescence to adulthood: an extension of theory and a review of research. Dev Psychol 1982;18:341-58.
[34] Chou C, Hsiao M C. Internet addiction, usage, gratifications, and pleasure experience—The Taiwan college students' case. Comput Educ 2000;35:65-80.
[35] Scherer K. College life online: healthy and unhealthy Internet use. J College Stud Dev 1997;38:655-65.
[36] Young KS. Internet addiction: the emergence of a new clinical disorder. Cyberpsychol Behav 1998;1:237-44.
[37] Asia Pacific Internet Research Alliance. Internet in Asia Pacific Region: a comparative report, 2008. Retrieved from: http://www.macaointernetproject.net/pdf/APIRA/Internet_in_Asia_Pacific_Region_20081225.pdf
[38] Nelson BV, Patience TH, MacDonald DC. Adolescent risk behavior and the influence of parents and education. J Am Board Fam Pract 1999;12:436-443.
[39] Shek DTL. Intact and non-intact families in Hong Kong: differences in perceived parental control processes, parent-child relational qualities, and adolescent psychological well-being. J Divorce Remarriage 2007;47:157-172.
[40] Shek DTL. Perceived parental control processes, parent-child relational qualities, and adolescent psychological well-being in intact and non-intact families: longitudinal findings in the Chinese culture. J Divorce Remarriage 2008:49:171-189.
[41] Catalano RF, Berglund ML, Ryan JAM, Lonczak HS, Hawkins JD. Positive youth development in the United States: research findings on evaluations of positive youth development programs. Prev Treat 2002;5:1-111.
[42] Fergus S, Zimmerman MA. Adolescent resilience: a framework for understanding healthy development. Annu Rev Public Health 2005;26:399-419.
[43] Shek DTL, Ma HK, editors. Special Issue: evaluation of the Project P.A.T.H.S.: replications. ScientificWorldJournal 2010;10:178-272.
[44] Wong FKD, Yan P, Lo E, Hung M. Mental health and social competence of mainland Chinese immigrant and local youth in Hong Kong: a comparison. J Ethnic Cultur Divers Soc Work 2003;12:85-110.
[45] Shek DTL, Ng CSM. Early identification of adolescents with greater psychosocial needs: an evaluation of the Project P.A.T.H.S. in Hong Kong. Int J Dis Hum Dev 2010;9:291-99.
[46] Shek DTL, Ng CSM, Tsui PF. Qualitative evaluation of the project P.A.T.H.S.: findings based on focus groups. Int J Dis Hum Dev 2010;9:307-13.
[47] Shek DTL, Yu L. A review of validated youth prevention and positive youth development programmes in Asia. Int J Adolesc Med Health 2011;23:317-24.
[48] Shek DTL. Quality of life of Chinese people in a changing world. Soc Indic Res 2010;95:357-61.
[49] Shek DTL. Quality of life research: responses to emerging issues in a changing world. Soc Indic Res 2011;100:371-74.

In: Adolescence and Behavior Issues in a Chinese Context ISBN: 978-1-62618-614-9
Editors: DTL Shek, RCF Sun and Joav Merrick

Chapter 5

CONSUMPTION OF PORNOGRAPHIC MATERIALS AMONG EARLY ADOLESCENTS IN HONG KONG

Daniel TL Shek, PhD, FHKPS, BBS, JP [*,1,2,3,4,5]
and Cecilia MS Ma, PhD [1]
[1]Department of Applied Social Sciences,
The Hong Kong Polytechnic University, Hong Kong, PRC
[2]Public Policy Research Institute,
The Hong Kong Polytechnic University, Hong Kong, PRC
[3]Department of Social Work, East China Normal University,
Shanghai, PRC
[4]Kiang Wu Nursing College of Macau, Macau, PRC
[5]Division of Adolescent Medicine, Department of Pediatrics,
Kentucky Children's Hospital, University of Kentucky,
College of Medicine, KY, US

ABSTRACT

This chapter looks at the consumption of pornographic materials by 3,328 Secondary 1 students in Hong Kong. Results showed that over 90% of the respondents had never consumed pornographic materials in the past year. Compared to traditional pornography, Internet pornography was the most common medium that participants used when viewing pornographic materials. Males reported a higher level of pornography exposure than females did. Results showed that different measures of positive youth development and family functioning were related to adolescents' consumption of pornographic materials. In general, higher levels of positive youth development and better family functioning were related to a lower level of pornography consumption. The relative contribution of positive youth development and family factors to consumption of pornographic materials was also explored.

---

[*] Correspondence: Professor Daniel T.L. Shek, PhD, FHKPS, BBS, JP, Chair Professor of Applied Social Sciences, Faculty of Health and Social Sciences, Department of Applied Social Sciences, The Hong Kong Polytechnic University, Room HJ407, Core H, Hunghom, Hong Kong. E-mail: daniel.shek@polyu.edu.hk.

INTRODUCTION

There are increasing concerns regarding the effects of sexualized media on the psychosexual development of adolescents. Sexual curiosity is the major reason for consumption of pornography among adolescents (1,2).

Studies showed that mass media were the most important source of sexual information among adolescents and young adults (3-6). In view of the proliferation of sexually explicit materials, Fisher and Barak (7) suggested that future research should focus on "a) personality characteristics that incline individuals to seek out sexually explicit materials…b) the effects of contact with sexually explicit media on individuals who chose to consume such material" (p. 315). It is noteworthy that previous studies mainly focused on the effects of pornography exposure among late adolescents and young adults (8-11) and there is not much research on consumption of pornographic materials in early adolescents. Hence, it is important to address this research gap.

Researchers argued that early exposure to pornography during adolescence might be associated with negative developmental outcomes, such as premarital sexual permissiveness, promiscuous sexual activity, sexually compulsive behavior and distorted belief of sexual activity (1,12-14). When adolescents were asked to recall their first exposure to sexual medium, negative emotions and physical responses (i.e., disgust, shock, embarrassment, anger, crying, sadness, guilt and confusion) were reported, and these results were more salient for 12-year-olds or younger (15). Past research investigating the influence of sexually explicit materials mainly examined traditional print pornography, with very few focusing on the potential harms of Internet pornography. Mental health practitioners and researchers viewed this new medium, which is extremely popular among adolescents, as a growing menace. This might be related to the easy accessibility, affordability and anonymity of the Internet (1). Adolescents often use the Internet for non-recreational (e.g., doing homework and project) and recreational purposes (e.g., playing online video games, watching videos, visiting social networking sites). Given that the Internet becomes an integral part of adolescents' life, factors related to online pornography exposure should be examined.

Similar to other places, there is an rising trend of Internet use in Hong Kong. Research findings showed that the percentage of Internet users rose from 40% in 2000 to 69% in 2008, in which Internet use among young adults (aged from 18-30 years) grew from 70% in 2000 to 98% in 2008 (16).

According to the statistics of the Hong Kong Census (17), the rates of Internet use among early adolescents (aged from 10-14 years) have remarkably increased (i.e., 73% in 2000 to 99% in 2009). The prevalence of Internet use was also supported by the increasing amount of online hours per week among Chinese adolescents (18,19). Prolonged Internet usage is susceptible to greater risk of Internet addiction. This is supported by a study of 6,121 Chinese middle and high school students where about 20% of the respondents were at risk for Internet addiction (19). Furthermore, Shek et al. (16) found that the frequency of leisure-time activities replacing Internet activities was a significant predictor of Internet addiction. The negative consequences of Internet addiction were invariant across cultures. As the Internet becomes more pervasive and popular among adolescents, identifying factors related to this type of pornographic materials would help us reduce its impact among Hong Kong adolescents in the future.

As the existing literature on consumption of pornographic materials is mainly based on Western populations, nothing is known about the pattern of pornography consumption and factors related to this behavior in Chinese contexts. Against this background, there are two purposes of this paper. First, descriptive profiles on pornographic material consumption in early Chinese adolescents are reported. Second, findings on the relationships between psychosocial correlates (including basic demographic factors, positive youth development qualities and family functioning) and exposure to traditional and Internet pornography in Hong Kong are presented.

OUR STUDY

The data reported in this paper were derived from the first wave of a six-year longitudinal study of adolescent development and their families in Hong Kong. The longitudinal study is a component of the extension phase of the Project P.A.T.H.S. which is financially supported by The Hong Kong Jockey Club Charities Trust.

A total of 3,328 Secondary 1 students (Grade 7) from 28 schools participated in this study. Among the participants, 1,719 (52%) were boys and 1,572 (48%) were girls, with 37 of them did not respond to the question. The mean age of the participants was 12.6 years old (*SD*=.74). The demographic information of the participants is shown in Table 1.

During data collection, the purpose of the study was mentioned and confidentiality of the collected data was repeatedly emphasized to all students in attendance on the day of testing. School, parental and student consent had been obtained prior to data collection.

Table 1. Demographic information of the respondents (*N*=3,328)

	n	%
Gender		
Male	1,719	52
Female	1,572	48
Place of birth		
Hong Kong	2,590	78
Mainland China	655	20
Others	64	2
Location of schools		
Hong Kong Island	5	18
Kowloon	7	25
New Territories	16	57
Parents' employment status		
Both parents were employed	1,643	57
Either father/mother was employed	956	33
Both parents were unemployed	305	11
Receiving financial aids		
Yes	225	7
No	2,606	79
Others	465	14

All participants responded to all scales in the questionnaire in a self-administration format. Adequate time was provided for the participants to complete the questionnaire. A trained research assistant was present throughout the administration process.

Instruments

The Chinese Positive Youth Development Scale (CPYDS)

The Chinese Positive Youth Development Scale (CPYDS) (20) was developed to assess positive youth development. The CPYDS has 15 subscales, including bonding (BO), resilience (RE), social competence (SC), recognition for positive behavior (PB), emotional competence (EC), cognitive competence (CC), behavioral competence (BC), moral competence (MC), self-determination (SD), self-efficacy (SE), clear and positive identity (SI), beliefs in the future (BF), prosocial involvement (PI), prosocial norms (PN) and spirituality (SP). The details of the items can be seen in Shek et al. (20). A 6-point Likert scale (1=strongly disagree to 6=strongly agree) was used to assess the responses of the participants. Using multigroup confirmatory factor analyses (MCFA), Shek and Ma (21) showed that the 15 basic dimensions of the CPYDS could be subsumed under four higher-order factors, including cognitive-behavioral competencies (CBC), prosocial attributes (PA), positive identity (PID) and general positive youth development qualities (GPYDQ). Evidence of factorial invariance in terms of configuration, first-order factor loadings, second-order factor loadings, intercepts of measured variable, and intercepts of first-order latent factor, was found. In short, existing research findings showed that the CPYDS is a valid and reliable instrument.

The Chinese Family Assessment Instrument (CFAI)

The Chinese Family Assessment Instrument (CFAI) was used to assess family functioning. In the present study, three subscales, including mutuality (mutual support, love and concern among family members), communication (frequency and nature of interaction among family members), conflicts and harmony (presence of conflicts and harmonious behavior in the family) were examined. The five response options were "very similar," "somewhat similar," "neither similar nor dissimilar," "somewhat dissimilar," and "very dissimilar." A higher total score on the subscales indicated a higher level of positive family functioning.

The reliability and validity of the CFAI were supported in previous studies (22-25). Furthermore, multigroup confirmatory factor analyses (MCFA) showed the existence of two higher-order factors (i.e., family interaction and parenting) and factorial invariance of the CFAI across gender and subgroups (26).

Exposure to pornographic materials

Twelve items were used to assess the consumption of two types of pornographic materials during the last year. They were Internet pornography (e.g., pornographic stories, pictures, videos and websites) and traditional pornography (e.g., pornographic movies, rental films, movies on cable TV, magazines, books and comics). Participants answered on a 6-point Likert-scale (0 = never; 1 = less than 1 time a month; 2 = 1-3 times a month; 3 = about 1 time a week; 4 = several times a week; 5 = daily).

Table 2. Past year exposure to Internet and traditional pornographic materials

	Never (%)	Less than 1 time a month (%)	1-3 times a month (%)	About 1 time a week (%)	Several times a week (%)	Daily (%)
Internet						
Pornographic stories	94.1	4.4	.8	.2	.4	.2
Pornographic pictures (exposed genitals)	93.0	5.6	.8	.2	.3	.1
Pornographic videos (exposed genitals)	93.7	4.4	1.0	.3	.4	.1
Sexual intercourse pictures (including comics)	93.6	4.4	1.1	.3	.4	.2
Sexual intercourse videos (including cartoons)	93.3	4.6	1.0	.4	.5	.1
Pornographic website	95.2	3.5	.8	.4	.1	.1
Traditional						
Pornographic movies	99.2	.6	.1	.0	.0	.0
Pornographic rental films	99.5	.3	.0	.1	.0	.0
Pornographic movies on cable TV	98.3	1.4	.1	.0	.1	.0
Pornographic magazines	98.7	.9	.2	.1	.1	.1
Pornographic books	98.6	1.0	.1	.1	.1	.1
Pornographic comics	97.1	2.1	.4	.2	.1	.1

Table 3. Past year exposure to Internet and traditional pornographic materials by gender

	Never (%)		Attempted (%)	
Internet	Male	Female	Male	Female
Pornographic stories	93.6	94.8	6.4	5.2
Pornographic pictures (exposed genitals)	90.6	95.7	9.4	4.3
Pornographic videos (exposed genitals)	91.0	96.9	9.0	3.1
Sexual intercourse pictures (including comics)	92.3	95.2	7.7	4.8
Sexual intercourse videos (including cartoons)	91.4	95.6	8.6	4.4
Pornographic website	92.6	98.0	7.4	2.0
Traditional				
Pornographic movies	98.7	99.9	1.3	.1
Pornographic rental films	99.3	99.8	.7	.2
Pornographic movies on cable TV	97.5	99.2	2.5	.8
Pornographic magazines	98.3	99.2	1.7	.8
Pornographic books	98.4	98.9	1.6	1.1
Pornographic comics	97.3	97.0	2.7	3.0

A composite score was calculated by averaging all twelve item scores in order to obtain the mean of the overall exposure to pornographic materials. The same method was used to calculate the mean consumption scores of traditional and Internet pornographic materials.

Family background characteristics

An item was asked to assess whether participants received financial aids (known as CSSA-comprehensive social security assistance) from the government of Hong Kong. For example *"Your family is now receiving CSSA?"* (1=Yes, 0=No). Another item was used to assess the immigrant status of the participants (0=Hong Kong, 1=mainland China, 2=others).

Perceived academic and school performance

Three items were tested to examine participants' perceptions on their academic and school competence. For example, "*Compared to your classmates, you think your academic performance is...?*", "*Are you satisfied with your academic results?*", "*You perceive your school conduct is...?*" There are five response options ("very bad", "bad", "average", "good", "very good"). A composite score was calculated by averaging all item scores in order to obtain the mean of the overall academic and school competence (ASC).

OUR FINDINGS

Reliability analyses showed that all subscales had acceptable internal consistency (Table 4). The prevalence of pornography consumption among Hong Kong adolescents is shown in Tables 2 and 3. Over 90% of adolescents reported they had never consumed pornographic materials over the past year. Compared to the traditional pornographic materials (mean rank=111.18), the degree of adolescents' exposure to the Internet pornographic materials was significantly higher (mean rank=223.87, $Z = -16.19$, $p < .01$).

Significant differences were found in gender and immigrant status, but not in family economic background (Table 5). Males (mean rank=1707.02) had a higher level of pornography consumption than females (mean rank=1579.28, $U = -6.41$, $p < .01$). Participants who were born in mainland China (mean rank=1729.47) reported a higher level of pornography consumption than those who were born in Hong Kong did (mean rank=1637.92, $U = -3.78$, $p < .01$). It is noteworthy that these differences were consistent in different types of pornographic materials. Analyses based on Pearson correlation showed that all positive youth development and family functioning measures were negatively correlated (ranging from -.06 to -.19) with the overall pornography exposure. In general, higher levels of positive youth development and family functioning were related to lower levels of pornography consumption (Table 4). To further examine the influence of individual and family background characteristics (i.e., age, gender, immigrant status, socioeconomic background) on the consumption of pornographic materials, multiple regression analyses were performed with individual and family factors as the predictors and different types of pornographic materials as the criterion variables. The findings based on multiple regression analyses can be seen in Table 6. Age, gender and immigrant status were significant predictors on pornographic materials. Results showed that higher levels of pornography exposure were found in older male participants, especially those who were born in mainland China. Also, results revealed that general positive youth development qualities second-order factor (GPYDQ), prosocial attributes second-order factor (PA) and family mutuality negatively predicted overall pornography exposure. However, it is noteworthy that cognitive-behavioral competencies second-order factor (CBC) and positive identity second-order factor (PID) positively predicted past year pornography exposure. Overall speaking, both positive youth development and family functioning negatively predicted adolescents' pornography consumption.

DISCUSSION

The goal of the current study was to examine the prevalence and psychosocial correlates of pornography consumption among Hong Kong Chinese early adolescents. There are several unique characteristics of the present study. First, in view of the paucity of pornography research in non-western contexts, a large Chinese sample was employed to provide a broader and comprehensive understanding of pornography consumption in different cultures. In fact, this is the first known scientific study of consumption of pornographic materials in different Chinese contexts. Second, two validated measures of positive youth development and family functioning in the Chinese contexts were used. Given the majority of this research area was conducted in Western countries, this study adds to the growing literature on pornography consumption. It sheds light on adolescent consumption of pornography and design of appropriate program for Chinese adolescents.

More than 90% of the participants reported that they had never read or watch pornographic materials in the past 12 months. These results were generally lower than those shown in Western populations (27-29). Given the younger age of the present study population, it is no surprise that the prevalence of pornography exposure was lower than those found in past research. In addition, sexual inhibition in the Chinese culture may also account for the findings.

Focusing exclusively on early adolescents, the present study extended past research by exploring whether the correlates of pornography consumption would vary by the types of pornographic materials—traditional and Internet pornography. Results showed that early adolescents consumed pornographic materials mostly from the Internet. As there are few studies comparing Internet-based versus traditional media in the consumption for pornographic materials, the current study is a pioneering work in pornography research.

In line with Western and Asian countries (9,11,30,31), the present study showed that Chinese males reported a higher degree of pornography exposure than Chinese females did, regardless of the types of pornographic materials. These findings highlighted the importance of providing help for adolescents, particularly males, regarding the consumption of pornographic materials. Males were more sexually exciting and likely to engage in sexual aggression than females after consuming pornographic materials (32,33). This is further supported by a study based on a sample of Chinese male young adults. Lam and Chan (10) found that repeated exposure to Internet pornography was associated with premarital sexual permissiveness and sexual harassment proclivity. Regarding the effects of pornography exposure, a comprehensive sex education program that addresses appropriate attitudes and values of sexual behavior is needed. It is noteworthy that in the extension phase of the Project P.A.T.H.S., new teaching units on sex education are designed.

Table 4. Descriptive statistics, internal consistencies and correlations among variables

	M (SD)	α (mean)[#]	Overall pornography (α=.91) r	Internet pornography (α=.92) r	Traditional pornography (α=.86) r
ASC	3.12 (.67)	.67 (.40)	-.06**	-.07**	-.02
Positive youth development					
CBC	4.45 (.75)	.82 (.61)	-.09**	-.09**	-.07**
PA	4.50 (.89)	.74 (.59)	-.19**	-.19**	-.15**
GPYDQ	4.58 (.71)	.88 (.48)	-.17**	-.16**	-.14**
PID	4.24 (.96)	.82 (.69)	-.09**	-.09**	-.08**
Family functioning					
Mutuality	3.89 (.89)	.87 (.70)	-.13**	-.12**	-.10**
Harmony	3.81 (.92)	.76 (.51)	-.11**	-.10**	-.08**
Communication	3.51 (1.01)	.81 (.59)	-.11**	-.11**	-.09**

Note. ASC: Academic and school competence; CBC: cognitive-behavioral competencies second-order factor; PA: prosocial attributes second-order factor; GPYDQ: general positive youth development qualities second-order factor; PID: positive identity second-order factor.

**$p < .01$. [#] Mean inter-item correlations.

Table 5. Mean rank differences among different types of pornographic materials by gender, immigrant status and family economic background

	Overall pornography		Internet pornography		Traditional pornography	
	Mean[#]	U	Mean[#]	U	Mean[#]	U
Gender						
Male	1707.02	-6.41**	1687.70	-6.50**	1640.83	-1.99**
Female	1579.28		1562.97		1616.13	
Immigrant status						
Hong Kong	1637.92	-3.78**	1619.67	-3.88**	1636.55	-.90
Mainland China	1729.47		1710.34		1649.98	
Receiving financial aids						
No	1413.70	-.67	1397.44	-.41	1399.68	-1.09
Yes	1436.33		1410.91		1422.94	

**$p < .01$. [#] Mean rank.

Table 6. Regression analyses based on individual- and family-related factors

Predictor	Overall pornography			Internet pornography			Traditional pornography		
	R	R^2	β^a	R	R^2	β^a	R	R^2	β^a
Block 1:									
Age			.04*			.05**			
Gender[1]			-.09**			-.11**			-.04*
Model	.10	.01		.12	.01		.04	.002	
Block 2:									
Immigrant status[#]			.04*			.05*			
Family economic status[^]									
Model	.06	.003		.06	.003		.04	.002	
Block 3:									
ASC									
Family functioning									
Mutuality			-.07*			-.07*			
Harmony									
Communication									
Positive youth development									
CBC			.08*						.10**
PA			-.17**			-.17**			-.12**
GPYDQ			-.10**			-.09*			-.10*
PID						.08*			
Model	.22	.05		.21	.05		.18	.03	

Note. ASC: Academic and school competence; CBC: cognitive-behavioral competencies second-order factor; PA: prosocial attributes second-order factor; GPYDQ: general positive youth development qualities second-order factor; PID: positive identity second-order factor.

[a] Standardized coefficients.

[1] Gender (0=male; 1=female).

[#] Immigrant status (only two levels were examined, i.e., 0=Hong Kong, 1=mainland China).

[^] Receiving financial aids (0=no; 1=yes). *$p < .05$, **$p < .01$.

Similar to Korean adolescents, negative relationships were shown between problem behaviors and psychological factors (30). These inverse relationships between positive youth development qualities and the degree of exposure to pornographic materials supported the notion that higher level of positive youth development qualities would predict lower level of youth health risk behaviors (34,35). In particular, prosocial attributes second-order factor and general positively youth development qualities second-order factor negatively predicted exposure to pornographic materials. This might be related to the conservative views towards sexuality and low prevalence of early sexual behaviors in Hong Kong (36,37). It is important to note that some positive youth developmental qualities were positively related to consumption of pornographic materials. One possibility is that young people with better cognitive competence and positive identity may over-estimate their self-control ability, thus attempting to explore pornographic materials. Also, higher social competence may induce peer support for the consumption of pornographic materials.

Research findings based on quantitative and qualitative research showed that pornography consumption can lead to normalization of sexual behavior and increasing likelihood of engaging in high-risk sexual activities, such as having multiple sexual partners, infections and pregnancy (32,38-40). Adolescents exposed to the sexually explicit materials would likely to be sexually inspired by the sexual content, motivate to experiment different sex acts, and thus affect their actual sex life (41).

Under the influence of this socializing effect, adolescents might follow a norm of relationship sex and have exaggerated and distorted beliefs of sexual activity among peers (40,42). To help adolescents aware the potential impact of this exposure, practitioners, parents, teachers should work together to educate them to obtain reliable health information, especially on the Internet, and to establish an honest and open discussion about responsible sexual behavior. This is paramount important as a study by Fok (43) showed that Hong Kong students perceived a discrepancy between the actual and expected sex education programs that were implemented in their schools. Therefore, educators should put more effort in promoting correct sex attitudes and values among Hong Kong adolescents.

In line with previous findings (44), family mutuality was a significant predictor to the consumption of pornographic materials. These findings further supported the beneficial effects of moral competence on reducing adolescents' pornography exposure with the presence of an open family communication atmosphere (45).

Contrary to our expectations, socioeconomic status failed to predict this problem behavior. Perhaps, other family related factors, such as parental control, satisfaction of parent-child relationship, should also be added to unravel the complex relationships among these variables in the future. In addition, financial hardship may also restraint the availability of pornographic materials in adolescents experiencing economic disadvantage.

Another factor that should be examined in future studies is whether the consumption of pornography is voluntary or not. Researchers noted that the possibility of inadvertent and unintentional exposure to pornography, especially in the peer-to-peer file-sharing network that serves as a popular means of downloading music and videos (46,47). Based on a sample of 1,500 young Internet users aged 10 to 17 years old, about 66% reported that they encountered unwanted exposed to pornography when surfing the Internet (48). Deliberate pornography was associated with high-risk sexual behaviors and detrimental to reproductive health (33,49,50).

Previous studies demonstrated that the adverse effects of unwanted exposure were more salient for youth with vulnerable characteristics, such as depression, offline interpersonal victimization (48). Future research should be conducted to solicit the information about their reason for visitation of sexual materials.

Also, other significant factors related to pornography exposure were not examined in the present study. For example, it would be interesting to test the relationship between exposure to pornographic materials and sexual behaviors. It seems that adolescents are more sexually aroused after reading or watching sexually explicit materials, and therefore would be likely to engage in sexual behaviors. This is supported by studies showing the positive association between exposure to Internet pornography and high-risk sexual behaviors among adolescents (13,51) and adults (52). Similar results were also found in a sample of Taiwanese adolescents (49). More work is needed to explore the impact of pornography exposure on adolescents' attitudes towards sexual behaviors in the future.

Several limitations of the current study must be noted. First, our study is based on respondents' self-report. Although anonymity and confidentiality were maintained in this study, social-desirability and other bias cannot not be eliminated. Second, as the present findings are based on Hong Kong adolescents, caution should be taken when generalized to other Chinese cultures, such as mainland China and Taiwan. Third, cross-sectional design of the study might rule out the causal relationship of the variables under investigation. More research should be conducted to examine the developmental effects of these psychological correlates among adolescents. This notion is reinforced by the recent findings which demonstrated that positive youth development programs such as the Project P.A.T.H.S. can help to reduce their negative behaviors among Hong Kong adolescents (53,54).

Despite the above limitations, the present study shows the important linkages between positive youth development qualities and pornography consumption among Hong Kong early adolescents. More efforts in promoting media literacy among this specific population should be emphasized.

As Hald (28) argued, "future research (should) focus on these situational, interpersonal, interpersonal, and behavioral characteristics of pornography consumption in addition to actual prevalence rates of consumption in different cultures" (p. 584). Obviously, our findings represent a positive response to this request. The present study sheds light on addressing the issue of contemporary pornography among Hong Kong adolescents. One recommended strategy is to implement school-based positive youth development programs such as the Project P.A.T.H.S. in Hong Kong (55-57).

ACKNOWLEDGMENTS

The preparation for this paper and the Project P.A.T.H.S. were financially supported by The Hong Kong Jockey Club Charities Trust. This chapter is based upon a paper published in the International Journal on Disability and Human Development (Shek DTL, Ma CMS. Consumption of pornographic materials among early adolescents in Hong Kong. Int J Disabil Hum Dev 2012;11(2):143-50). Permission has been obtained from the publisher to publish this modified version of the paper in this book.

REFERENCES

[1] Cooper ML, Shaver PR, Collins NL. Attachment styles, emotion regulation and adjustment in adolescence. J Pers Soc Psychol 1998;74(5):1380-97.

[2] Goodson P, McCormick D, Evans A. Searching for sexually explicit materials on the Internet: An exploratory study of college students' behavior and attitudes. Arch Sex Behav 2001;30:101-8.

[3] Duncan, D. Pornography as a source of sex information for students at a private northeastern university. Psychol Rep 1991;68:782.

[4] Duncan DF, Nicholsson T. Pornography as a source of sex information for students at a southeastern state university. Psychol Rep 1991;68:802.

[5] Griffiths M. Excessive Internet use: Implications for sexual behavior. CyperPsychol 2000;3(4):537-52.

[6] Trostle L. Pornography as a source of sex information for university students: Some consistent findings. Psychol Rep 1993:72:407-12.

[7] Fisher WA, Barak A. Internet pornography: A social psychological perspective on internet sexuality. J Sex Res 2001;38:312-23.

[8] Fu KW, Chan, WSC, Wong PWC, Yip PSF. Internet addiction: Prevalence, discriminant validity and correlates among adolescents in Hong Kong. British J Psychiatry 2010;196;486-92.

[9] Janghorbani M, Lam TH, The Youth Sexuality Study Task Force. Sexual media use by young adults in Hong Kong: Prevalence and associated factors. Arch Sex Behav 2003;32:545-53.

[10] Lam CB, Chan DKS. The use of cyberpornography by young men in Hong Kong: Some psychosocial correlates. Arch Sex Behav 2007;36:588-98.

[11] Sabina C, Wolak J, Finkelhor D. The nature and dynamics of Internet pornography exposure for youth. CyberPsychol Behav 2008;11(6):691-3.

[12] Kanuga M, Rosenfeld WD. Adolescent sexuality and the Internet: The good, the bad, and the URL. J Pedia Adolesc Gynecol 2004;17:117-24.

[13] Malamuth N, Impett E. Research on sex in the media: What do we know about effects on children and adolescents? In: Singer DG, Singer J, eds. Handbook of children and the media. Thousand Oaks,CA: Sage, 2001:269-87.

[14] Rich M. Sex screen: The dilemma of media exposure and sexual behavior. Pediatrics 2007;116(1):329-31.

[15] Cantor J, Mares ML, Hyde JS. Autobiographical memories of exposure to sexual media content. Media Psychol 2003;5:1-31.

[16] Hong Kong Internet Project. Internet use in Hong Kong: The 2008 Annual survey report. Hong Kong: Hong Kong Internet Project, 2009.

[17] Hong Kong Census and Statistic Department. Usage of personal computers and internet services by Hong Kong residents, 2000 to 2009. Hong Kong: Census and Statistic Department, 2010.

[18] Ho SMY, Lee TMC. Computer usage and its relationship with adolescent lifestyle in Hong Kong. J Adoles Health 2001;29:258-66.

[19] Shek DTL, Tang VM, Lo CY. Internet addiction in Chinese adolescents in Hong Kong: Assessment, profiles, and psychosocial correlates. ScientificWorldJounral 2008;8:776-87.

[20] Shek DTL, Siu AMH, Lee TY. The Chinese positive youth development Scale: A validation study. Res Soc Work Pract 2007;12(3):380-91.

[21] Shek DTL, Ma CMS. Dimensionality of the Chinese Positive Youth Development Scale: confirmatory factor analyses. Soc Indic Res 2010;98:41-59.

[22] Shek DTL. Assessment of family functioning: The Chinese version of the Family Assessment Device. Res Soc Work Prac 2002;12:502-24.

[23] Shek DTL. Assessment of family functioning Chinese adolescents: The Chinese Family Assessment Instrument. In: Singh NN, Ollen-dick T, Singh AN, eds. International perspectives on child and adolescent mental health. Amsterdam: Elsevier, 2002:297-316.

[24] Siu AMH, Shek DTL. Psychometric properties of the Chinese Family Assessment Instrument in Chinese adolescents in Hong Kong. Adolesc 2005;40:817-30.

[25] Shek DTL. Family functioning and psychological well-being, school adjustment, and substance abuse in Chinese adolescents: Are findings based on multiple studies consistent? In: Shohov SP, ed. Advances in psychology research. New York: Nova Science, 2003:163-84.

[26] Shek DTL, Ma CMS. The Chinese Family Assessment Instrument (C-FAI): Hierarchical confirmatory factor analyses and factorial invariance. Res Soc Work Pract 2010;20(1):112-23.

[27] Braun-Courville DK, Rojas M. Exposure to sexually explicit web sites and adolescent sexual attitudes and behaviors. J Adolesc Health 2009;45:156-62.

[28] Hald GM. Gender differences in pornography consumption among young heterosexual Danish adults. Arch Sex Beahv 2006;35:577-85.

[29] Peter J, Valkenburg M. The use of sexually explicit Internet material and its antecedents: A longitudinal comparison of adolescents and adults. Arch Sex Behav 2010. doi: 10.1007/s10508-010-9644-x

[30] Kim YH. Korean Adolescetns' health risk behaviors and their relationships with the selected psychological constructs. 2001;29:298-306.

[31] Svedin CG, Åkerman I, Priebe G. Frequent users of pornography: A population based epidemiological study of Swedish male adolescents. J Adolesc, 2010. doi:10.1016/j.adolescence.2010.04.010

[32] Traeen B, Sorheim-Nielsen T, Beverfjord A. Attitudes and use of pornography in the Norwegian population 2002. J Sex Res 2004;41:193-200.

[33] Zillmann D. Influence of unrestrained access to erotica on adolescents' and young adults' dispositions toward sexuality. J Adolesc Health 2000;27:41-4.

[34] Catalano RF, Berglund ML, Ryan JAM, Lonczak HS, Hawkins JD. Positive youth development in the United States: Research findings on evaluations of positive youth development programs. Prev Treat 2002;5:15.

[35] Gavin LE, Catalano RF, David-Ferdon C, Gloppen KM, Markham CM. A review of positive youth development programs that promote adolescent sexual and reproductive health. J Adolesc Health 2010;46:S75-91.

[36] Lam TH, Xenos PS, Au PK, Lee JMK, Lee PWH, Ng ML et al. Report on youth sexuality study (Form 3-7 student survey). Hong Kong: The Family Planning Association of Hong Kong, 2000.

[37] Lam TH, Stewart SM, Ho LM. Smoking and high-risk sexual behavior among young adults in Hong Kong. J Behav Medicine 2001;24:503-16.

[38] Rubington E, Weinberg MS. Deviance: The interactionist perspective. Boston: Allyn and Bacon, 1996.

[39] Strasburger VC, Wilson BJ. Children, adolescents, and the media. Thousand Oaks, CA: Sage, 2002.

[40] Weinberg MS, Williams CJ, Kleiner S, Irizarry Y. Pornography, normalization, and empowerment. Arch Sex Behav 2010;39:1389-401.

[41] Štulhofer A, Buško V, Landripet I. Pornography, sexual socialization, and satisfaction among young men. Arch Sex Behav 2010;39(1):168-78.

[42] Paul P. Pornified: How pornography is transforming our lives, our relationships, and our families. New York: Holt, 2005.

[43] Fok SC. A study of the implementation of sex education in Hong Kong secondary schools. Sex Edu 2005;5(3):281-94.

[44] Kung EM, Farrell AD. The role of parents and peers in early adolescent substance use: An examination of mediating and moderating effects. J Child Fam Studies 2000;9:509-28.

[45] Bryant J, Rockwell SC. Effects of massive exposure to sexually oriented prime-time television on adolescents' moral judgmnet. In: Zillmann D, Bryant J, Huston AC, eds. Media, children, and the family. Hillsdale, NJ: Lawrence Erlbaum, 1994.

[46] Greenfield P. Developmental considerations for determining appropriate Internet use guidelines for children and adolectns. J App Develop Psychol 2004;25:751-62.

[47] Thornburgh D, Lin HS. Committee to study tools and strategies for protecting kids from pornography and their applicability to other Internet content. In: Thornburgh D, Lin HS, eds. Youth, pornography, and the Internet. Washington, DC: National Academy Press, 2002.

[48] Lo V, Wei R. Exposure to Internet pornography and Taiwanese adolescents' sexual attitudes and behavior. J Broadcast Electron Media 2005;49:221-37.

[49] Häggström-Nordin E, Hanson U, Tydén T. Associations between pornography consumption and sexual practices among adolescents in Sweden. Int J STD AIDS 2005;16:102-7.

[50] Wolak J, Mitchell K, Finkelhor D. Unwanted and wanted exposure to online pornography in a national sample of youth Internet users. Pediatrics 2007;119:247-57.

[51] Braun-Couville D, Rojas M. Exposure to sexually explicit web sites and adolescent sexual attitudes and behaviors. J Adolesc Health 2009;45:156-62.

[52] Rogal C, Tyden T. Does pornography influence young women's sexual behavior? Women's Health Issues 2003;13:39-43.

[53] Shek DTL, Ma CMS. Impact of the Project P.A.T.H.S. in the junior secondary school years: Individual growth curve analyses. ScientificWorldJournal 2011;11:253-66.

[54] Shek DTL, Yu L. Prevention of Adolescent Problem Behavior: Longitudinal impact of the Project P.A.T.H.S. in Hong Kong ScientificWorldJournal 2011;11:546-87.

[55] Shek DTL, Ng CSM. Early identification of adolescents with greater psychosocial needs: An evaluation of the Project P.A.T.H.S. in Hong Kong. Int J Dis Hum Dev 2010;9:291-9.

[56] Shek DTL, Ng CSM, Tsui PF. Qualitative evaluation of the project P.A.T.H.S.: Findings based on focus groups. Int J Dis Hum Dev 2010;9:307-13.

[57] Shek, DTL. Quality of life of Chinese people in a changing world. Soc Indic Res 2010;95:357-61.

In: Adolescence and Behavior Issues in a Chinese Context ISBN: 978-1-62618-614-9
Editors: DTL Shek, RCF Sun and Joav Merrick

Chapter 6

DELINQUENCY AND PROBLEM BEHAVIOR INTENTION AMONG EARLY ADOLESCENTS IN HONG KONG

Daniel TL Shek, PhD, FHKPS, BBS, JP*[*1,2,3,4,5], and Cecilia MS Ma, PhD[1]

[1]Department of Applied Social Sciences,
The Hong Kong Polytechnic University, Hong Kong, PRC
[2]Public Policy Research Institute,
The Hong Kong Polytechnic University, Hong Kong, PRC
[3]Department of Social Work, East China Normal University, Shanghai, PRC
[4]Kiang Wu Nursing College of Macau, Macau, PRC
[5]Division of Adolescent Medicine, Department of Pediatrics,
Kentucky Children's Hospital, College of Medicine,
University of Kentucky, KY, US

ABSTRACT

Delinquency and problem behavior intention were examined in 3,328 Secondary One students in Hong Kong. Over 60% of the respondents had cheated and spoken foul language over the past year, but majority of them had never engaged in other problem behaviors, such as sexual intercourse, staying outside home overnight, gang fighting, and truancy. A significant proportions of the respondents would attempt to engage in delinquent behaviors in the coming two years, including drinking alcohol and gambling. Males reported higher levels of delinquency and problem behavior intention than did females. Higher family functioning, academic competence, prosocial attributes, and general positive youth development predicted a lower likelihood of delinquency and problem behavior intention. These results shed light on the importance of early intervention work at individual, school, and family levels.

---

* Correspondence: Professor Daniel T.L. Shek, PhD, FHKPS, BBS, JP, Chair Professor of Applied Social Sciences, Department of Applied Social Sciences, The Hong Kong Polytechnic University, Hunghom, Hong Kong, P.R.C. E-mail: daniel.shek@polyu.edu.hk.

INTRODUCTION

During adolescence, young people have to face both physiological and psychological changes, search for self-identity, and struggle for independence. Hall (1,2) described this stage as "storm and stress". Facing these developmental changes, there is a tendency for adolescents to have conflicts with their parents, disrupted moods, and increased propensity for reckless and problem behavior (2). Youth problem behavior can be regarded as a part of the growth process or an indicator of a long-term trend of criminal activity (2). In view of its potential harmful impacts on the individual, family, and community, intervention is necessary to support adolescents before problem behavior occurs. Through the examination of prevalence and psychosocial correlates of youth problem behavior, youth programs that address risk and protective factors in delinquency could be developed.

Problem behavior theory is commonly used to understand the nature and development of youth problem behavior (3). This theory encompasses three major dimensions of the individual system: an individual's personality, perceived environment, and behavior. The likelihood of occurrence of problem behavior is specified by the proneness of each dimension, a dynamic state reflecting either instigations to problem behavior or controls against it (3). The personality dimension includes a set of personal characteristics, such as value on achievement and self-esteem. The perceived environment dimension refers to the proximal and distal social influence factors such as family and peer orientation and expectations regarding problem behavior. The behavior dimension consists of the degree of involvement in other problem behaviors and conventional behaviors (such as church and school attendance).

Many researchers have used the problem behavior theoretical framework to examine youth delinquency. In the personality dimension, researchers found that low self-esteem, hopelessness, low sense of mastery, avoidance coping, aggression, and impulsivity were associated with youth problem behavior (4-6). In particular, Barber (5) pointed out that externalizing personality traits like aggression, impulsivity, and rebelliousness were related to externalizing problems like substance use and delinquency, while more internalizing personality characteristics like social isolation, hopelessness, and self-hatred were associated with internalizing problems such as depression, suicide, and eating disorders. In the perceived environment dimension, family is regarded as "the single influential childhood factor in buffering the child and in shaping later adaptation" (p. 22) (7).

Western studies showed a wide range of adverse family conditions, such as lack of parental supervision, low parental attachment, poor parenting practice, parents' deviant behavior and attitude, and parental separation, were related to youth problem behavior (8). This is further supported by a study which showed that students with well supervision and support from parents would be less likely to engage in problem behavior than their counterparts under adverse family conditions (9).

Lastly, in the behavior dimension, numerous studies revealed that lack of school bonding or school dropout was strongly correlated with problem behavior (4,10). Eccles (10) asserted that age-related increase in such negative motivational and behavioral characteristics such as test anxiety, learned helplessness, truancy, and school dropout made some adolescents prone to problem behavior. To delay the onset of delinquency, it is important to understand the prevalence as well as risk and protective factors of problem behavior in early adolescence.

Besides, previous studies mainly focused on examining psychosocial factors of students' past problem behavior. Several social-psychological models (e.g., theory of reasoned action, theory of planned behavior, and protection motivation theory) have highlighted an individual's intention to perform certain behavior as an important predictor to actual behavior (11-13). Against this background, researchers began to investigate the role of behavioral intention in adolescent problem behaviors such as sex and drug use (14-16). However, there is a paucity of research examining the relationship between problem behavior intention and psychosocial correlates of youth delinquency.

Despite the vast literature on adolescent risk behavior in the West, there are comparatively fewer studies in Chinese contexts. In Hong Kong, the patterns of youth problem behaviors such as smoking, substance abuse, physical violence, sexual activity, and gambling were examined (17-23). Similar to Western studies (4,9,10), there was age-related increase in delinquency (20,21). Also, the findings were related to the three dimensions of the problem behavior theory. In the personality dimension, poor psychosocial competencies, lower life satisfaction, and poor self-concept were correlated with problem behavior (21-23).

In the perceived environment dimension, studies (18,21,24) found that adolescents with a more negative family environment, including negative parenting styles, poor family functioning, lesser family involvement, more parent-child conflicts, and family violence, reported more problem behaviors. In the behavior dimension, youth problem behavior was indicated by their negative perception of school and examination pressure, academic performance, teachers and classmates (18,21). Specifically, lack of school bonding predicted students' problem behavior at school (18). Compared with Western findings, Hong Kong adolescents appeared to report lower rates of problem behavior (17-21,25,26). These differences might be related to the stress of familism and academic achievement in the Chinese culture, which contribute to stronger buffers at family and school levels (27). As commented by Shek (24), emphasis of familism and harmony within the family in Chinese societies might reduce the negative impact of a poor family environment on adolescent development. Since academic performance was the most pressing concern to Hong Kong students (28-30), they might have stronger personal value on achievement and perhaps stronger school bonding, protecting them away from problem behavior. Therefore, it seems that Chinese societal norms of filial piety and academic achievement may provide Hong Kong adolescents with stronger protective power at personality, perceived environment, and behavior dimensions against delinquency. In view of the possible cultural differences on the influence of psychosocial correlates, more research in the Chinese context is needed. There are two objectives of this paper. First, descriptive profiles on delinquency and behavior intention to engage in problem behavior among Chinese Secondary One students are reported. Second, findings on the relationships between psychosocial correlates (including basic demographic factors, positive youth development qualities, family functioning, and academic competence) and delinquency and problem behavioral intention are presented.

OUR STUDY

The present study is part of a large longitudinal study aiming at tracking the developmental trends of different positive youth development indicators and risk behaviors among Hong

Kong adolescents over time. A total of 28 secondary schools in Hong Kong were randomly selected to participate in the study. Data regarding delinquency and problem behavior intention collected at Wave 1 are reported in this paper.

Participants

A total of 3,328 Secondary One students participated in the study. The mean age of the participants was 12.59 years (*SD* = 0.74). These included 1,719 boys, 1,572 girls, and 37 students did not indicate their gender. While most students were born in Hong Kong (78.1%), there were 19.9% of the participants from mainland China and 2.0% from other places. The demographic information of the participants is summarized in Table 1.

Table 1. Demographic information of the respondents (*N*=3,328)

	n	%
Gender		
Male	1,719	52
Female	1,572	48
Place of birth		
Hong Kong	2,590	78
Mainland China	655	20
Others	64	2
School location		
Hong Kong Island	5	18
Kowloon	7	25
New Territories	16	57
Parents' marital status		
Divorced	209	6
Separated	73	2
First marriage	2,781	84
Second marriage	129	4
Others	104	3
Parents' employment status		
Both parents were employed	1,643	57
Either father/mother was employed	956	33
Both parents were unemployed	305	11
Receiving financial aids		
Yes	225	7
No	2,606	79
Others	465	14

Procedures

In the school year of 2009-2010, the participants were invited to respond to a comprehensive youth development questionnaire including both existing instruments and scales developed by the first author. The questionnaire survey was conducted by a trained research assistant in classroom settings with standardized instructions. At each measurement occasion, the purposes of the study were introduced and confidentiality of the data collected was repeatedly emphasized to all participants. School, parental, and student consent had been obtained before data collection. Participants responded to the questionnaires in a self-administered format. The research assistant was present throughout the administration process to answer possible questions from the participants.

Instruments

Participants were invited to respond to a composite questionnaire that comprised questions about demographic information, participants' family environment, different measures of youth development constructs and problem behavior. With reference to the objectives of this study, the scales used to assess delinquency, positive youth development, school adjustment and family socio-economic status are described below. Internal consistency of each measure and correlations among them are shown in Table 2.

Table 2. Descriptive statistics, internal consistencies, and correlations among variables

	M (SD)	α (mean)[#]	Delinquency *r*	Problem behavior intention *r*
Delinquency	.39 (.47)	.70 (.25)	-	.50**
Problem behavior intention	.26 (.39)	.64 (.36)	.50**	-
Academic and school competence	3.12 (.67)	.67 (.40)	-.21**	-.17**
Positive youth development				
CBC	4.45 (.75)	.82 (.61)	-.21**	-.15**
PA	4.50 (.89)	.74 (.59)	-.35**	-.25**
GPYDQ	4.58 (.71)	.88 (.48)	-.34**	-.26**
PIT	4.24 (.96)	.82 (.69)	-.23**	-.15**
Family functioning				
Mutuality	3.89 (.89)	.87 (.70)	-.29**	-.23**
Harmony	3.81 (.92)	.76 (.51)	-.25**	-.23**
Communication	3.51 (1.01)	.81 (.59)	-.31**	-.23**

Note. CBC: cognitive-behavioral competencies second-order factor; PA: prosocial attributes second-order factor; GPYDQ: general positive youth development qualities second-order factor; PIT: positive identity second-order factor.

** $p < .01$.

[#] Mean inter-item correlations.

Delinquency scale

This scale comprised 12 items that assessed the frequency of delinquent behaviors of the participants in the past one year, including stealing, cheating, truancy, running away from home, damaging others' properties, assault, having sexual intercourse with others, gang fighting, speaking foul language, staying outside the home overnight without parental consent, strong arming others, and trespasses (31). Respondents rated the frequency of these behaviors in the past one year on a six-point Likert scale (0 = never, 1 = one to two times; 2 = three to four times; 3 = five to six times; 4 = seven to eight times; 5 = nine to ten times; 6 = more than ten times).

Problem behavior intention scale

Five items were used to assess the participants' behavioral intention to engage in problem behaviors, including drinking alcohol, smoking, taking drugs (such as ketamine, cannabis, or ecstasy), having sex with others, and gambling. Respondents were asked to rate the likelihood that they may engage in these problem behaviors in the next two years on a four-point Likert scale, with "0" representing "never", "1" representing "not likely", "2" representing "likely", and "3" representing "definitely".

Chinese Positive Youth Development Scale (CPYDS)

The CPYDS consisted of 15 subscales which were listed as follows:

1. Bonding Subscale (three items)
2. Resilience Subscale (three items)
3. Social Competence Subscale (three items)
4. Emotional Competence Subscale (three items)
5. Cognitive Competence Subscale (three items)
6. Behavioral Competence Subscale (three items)
7. Moral Competence Subscale (three items)
8. Self-Determination Subscale (three items)
9. Self-Efficacy Subscale (two items)
10. Beliefs in the Future Subscale (three items)
11. Clear and Positive Identity Subscale (three items)
12. Spirituality Subscale (three items)
13. Prosocial Involvement Subscale (three items)
14. Prosocial Norms Subscale (three items)
15. Recognition for Positive Behavior Subscale (three items)

Based on factor analyses, Shek and Ma (32) proposed that the 15 subscales in the CPYDS could be further reduced to four dimensions:

1. Cognitive-Behavioral Competencies (CBC): Scale score was calculated by averaging scores on Cognitive Competence Subscale, Self-Determination Subscale, and Behavioral Competence Subscale.
2. Prosocial Attributes (PA): Scale score equaled to the mean score of Prosocial Involvement Subscale and Prosocial Norms Subscale.
3. Positive Identity (PIT): Scale score was computed by averaging scores of Beliefs in the Future Subscale and Clear and Positive Identity Subscale.
4. General Positive Youth Development Qualities (GPYDQ): Scale score equaled to the mean score of Resilience Subscale, Social Competence Subscale, Self-Efficacy Subscale, Moral Competence Subscale, Bonding Subscale, Recognition for Positive Behavior Subscale, Spirituality Subscale, and Emotional Competence Subscale.

Chinese Family Assessment Instrument (CFAI)

The Chinese Family Assessment Instrument (CFAI) was used to assess perceived family functioning. In the present study, three subscales, including mutuality (mutual support, love, and concern among family members), communication (frequency and nature of interaction among family members), conflicts and harmony (presence of conflicts and harmonious behavior in the family) were examined. The five response options were "very similar," "somewhat similar," "neither similar nor dissimilar," "somewhat dissimilar," and "very dissimilar." A higher total score on the subscales indicated a higher level of positive family functioning. The reliability and validity of the CFAI were supported in previous studies (33-36). Furthermore, multigroup confirmatory factor analyses (MCFA) showed the existence of two higher order factors (i.e., family interaction and parenting) and factorial invariance of the CFAI across genders and subgroups (37).

Academic and School Competence Scale (ASC)

As a relatively independent positive youth development construct, participants' academic and school competence (ASC) were measured by three items. For the first item, participants were required to rate their perceived academic performance as compared to other peer students on a five-point Likert scale, with "1" = "very poor", "2" = "below average", "3" = "average", "4" = "above average", and "5" = "very good". The second item asked the extent to which the respondents were satisfied with their academic performance ("1" = "very dissatisfied", "2" = "dissatisfied", "3" = "neutral", "4" = "satisfied", and "5" = "very satisfied"). The last question asked the participants to rate their conduct in school on a five-point Likert scale ("1" = "very poor", "2" = "below average", "3" = "average", "4" = "above average", and "5" = "very good"). The ASC scale score was calculated by averaging the item scores and ranged from 1 to 5, with high scores representing for high academic and school competence.

Data analytic plan

Descriptive analysis was run to show the picture of delinquency and problem behavior intention among Hong Kong early adolescents. Mann-Whitney *U* tests were used to examine gender and socio-economic differences on two dimensions. Further, to investigate whether gender, age, immigration status, family economic status, family functioning, academic and school competence, and positive youth development are predictive of adolescent delinquency and problem behavior intention, multiple regression analysis was performed. A total of fourteen independent variables were divided into five blocks for analysis. Students' basic demographic factors (i.e., age and gender) were entered in the first block; their socio-economic background variables (i.e., immigration status and family economic status) were entered in the second block; their family functioning, including family mutuality, communication, and harmony were entered into the third block; their personal psychosocial attributes (i.e., academic and school competence (ASC), cognitive-behavioral competencies (CBC), prosocial attributes (PA), positive identity (PIT), and general positive youth development qualities (GPYDQ)) were entered into the fourth block; their total scores of Chinese positive youth development and Chinese family functioning were entered into the fifth block of the regression model.

OUR FINDINGS

As shown in Table 3, smoking and speaking foul language were two popular delinquent behaviors that Secondary One students had exhibited over the year. Over 60% of the respondents had cheated and spoken foul language, of which around 12-25% had exhibited such behaviors seven times or above in the past year. Apart from these two behaviors, consistent with the prior literature, Hong Kong students' rate of delinquency was generally lower than their counterparts in the West (25,26). Over 84% of the respondents had never displayed any other delinquent behaviors. In particular, 99.3% of them had never had sexual intercourse with others. Similarly, the respondents had shown low intention to engage in problem behavior in the coming two years. Over 91% of students reported that they would not smoke, take drugs, and have sexual intercourse with others (Table 4). However, it should be noted that nearly one-third of the respondents showed intention to drink alcohol and around 8% of them would gamble.

Gender differences

Gender, immigration, and family economic statuses were examined with Mann-Whitney *U* Test. As shown in Table 5, significant differences were found in gender. Males (mean rank = 1597.12) had a higher level of delinquency than did females (mean rank =1484.15, $U = -3.55$, $p < .01$). Males (mean rank = 1680.82) also reported a higher level of problem behavior intention than did females (mean rank =1573.84, $U = -3.51$, $p < .01$).

Table 3. Percentage of respondents with delinquent behavior

Delinquent behavior in the past one year	Never (%)	1-6 times (%)	7 times or above (%)
1. Stealing	89.9	9.6	0.5
2. Cheating	39.2	48.4	12.4
3. Truancy	96.7	2.9	0.4
4. Running away from home	96.0	3.8	0.2
5. Damaging others' properties	86.5	12.6	0.8
6. Assault	88.3	10.3	1.4
7. Having sexual intercourse with others	99.3	0.6	0.1
8. Gang fighting	96.7	2.9	0.4
9. Speaking foul language	30.7	44.7	24.6
10. Staying outside the home overnight without parental consent	97.0	2.4	0.6
11. Strong arming others	84.4	13.3	2.3
12. Trespasses	96.2	3.4	0.3

$^{*}p < .05$; $^{**}p < .01$.

Table 4. Percentage of participants with intention to engage in problem behavior

Intention to engage in problem behavior in coming two years		Never (%)	Not likely (%)	Likely (%)	Definitely (%)
1.	Drinking alcohol	55.7	15.6	22.8	5.8
2.	Smoking	91.6	4.8	2.6	1.0
3.	Taking drugs	97.6	1.5	0.5	0.4
4.	Having sexual intercourse with others	93.5	4.1	1.8	0.6
5.	Gambling	82.8	8.9	6.3	2.0

$^{*}p < .05$; $^{**}p < .01$.

Correlates and predictors of delinquency and problem behavior intention

Analyses based on Pearson correlation showed that academic and school competence, positive youth development, and family functioning measures were all negatively correlated (ranging from -.15 to -.35) with delinquency and problem behavior intention. In general, higher levels of academic and school competence, positive youth development, and family functioning were related to lower levels of past and future problem behavior (Table 2).

Table 5. Mean rank differences among delinquency and problem behavior intention by gender, immigrant status and family economic status

	Delinquency		Problem behavior intention	
	Mean#	*U*	Mean#	*U*
Gender				
Male	1597.12	-3.55**	1680.82	-3.51**
Female	1484.15		1573.84	
Immigration status				
Hong Kong	1539.47	-1.61	1625.31	-1.93
Mainland China	1602.00		1696.41	
Receiving financial aids				
No	1319.78	-1.34	1405.83	-1.29
Yes	1393.70		1338.58	

$^{**}p < .01$.
Mean rank.

Regression analysis results are presented in Table 6. Age, gender, family harmony and communication, academic and school competence, as well as all positive youth development measures were significant predictors of both delinquency and problem behavior intention. Older and mainland immigrant males who had poor academic and school competence, family functioning, and psychosocial attributes would be likely to engage in problem behavior. Despite the significant results, all five models only accounted for 0-16% of past delinquency and 1-11% of future problem behavior intention. While students' socio-economic background predicted the least, their personal psychosocial attributes predicted the most. It is also noteworthy that cognitive-behavioral competencies second-order factor (CBC) and positive identity second-order factor (PIT) positively predicted students' delinquency and problem behavior intention.

Table 6. Regression analyses based on individual- and family-related factors

	Delinquency			Problem behavior intention		
Predictor	R	R^2	β^a	R	R^2	β^a
Age			.08**			.11**
Gender[Δ]			-.08**			-.06**
Model	.11	.01		.13	.02	
Immigration status[#]			.03			.07**
CSSA[^]			.01			-.03
Model	.03	.00		.07	.01	
Mutuality			-.06*			-.05
Harmony			-.11**			-.14**
Communication			-.21**			-.12**
Model	.33	.11		.27	.07	
ASC			-.09**			-.11**
CBC			.12**			.08**
PA			-.24**			-.17**
GPYDQ			-.30**			-.28**
PIT			.09**			.15**
Model	.40	.16		.32	.11	
CYPDS			-.23**			-.15**
CFAI			-.21**			-.19**
Model	.38	.14		.29	.09	

Note. ASC: academic and school competence; CBC: cognitive-behavioral competencies second-order factor; PA: prosocial attributes second-order factor; GPYDQ: general positive youth development qualities second-order factor; PIT: positive identity second-order factor; CYPDS: total score of positive youth development; CFAI: total score of Chinese family functioning.

[a] Standardized coefficients.

[Δ] Gender (0=male; 1=female).

[#] Immigration status (only two levels were examined, i.e., 0=Hong Kong, 1=mainland China).

[^] Receiving financial aids (0=no; 1=yes).

$*p < .05$, $**p < .01$.

Discussion

This paper presents findings on the descriptive profiles of delinquency and problem behavior intention among Hong Kong Secondary One students. Consistent with previous studies, Hong Kong adolescents reported lower rates of problem behavior than did their counterparts in the West (17-21,25,26). In particular, almost all of the students had never had sexual intercourse with others. The lower rate might be explained by the influence of a different socialization environment (38). Socialization interacts with developmental characteristics in adolescence might influence the types and rates of risk behavior undertaken within specific cultures. In regard to Chinese parenting and schooling which stress firm discipline and inhibition, Hong Kong students might have higher obedience, conformity, and respect for social order, therefore contributing to the lower rate of delinquency than their Western counterparts (27).

In line with both Western and local studies (17-21,25,26), the present findings showed that individual psychosocial attributes, family functioning, and academic and school competence were negatively related to youth delinquency and problem behavior intention. Compared with student demographic characteristics, all these psychosocial correlates together had higher predictive power of delinquency.

Hirschi (39) regarded social bonds in family and school as important sources of informal social control, which in turn reduces youth delinquency. Both family and school can contribute to the creation of social bond through the provision of internalized controls, indirect controls, direct controls, and need satisfaction (40). At the family level, local studies (18,21,24,40,41) consistently supported that good family functioning was negatively related to frequency of problem behavior. Since Chinese parenting is more controlling and restrictive than that of the West (40-42), strong family bonding would protect students from engaging in problem behavior. However, it should be noted that such controlling parenting style might contribute to lesser care and communication with children amongst Chinese parents (43). In this study, family communication was one important protective factor of delinquency. As adolescence is a stage for independence, it is recommended that parents provide more democratic communication, which emphasizes autonomy and self-direction of their children in response to their individual needs (44). Because family influences on children might decline with age (6), family intervention work should be started as early as possible to buffer and shape their later adaptation.

At the school level, this study supported previous findings that poor academic performance was related to students' problem behavior (4,8,18,21,40). Academic achievement is long perceived in Chinese culture to bring about economic and social advancement as well as moral development (18). It is even regarded as the most pressing concern among Hong Kong adolescents (28). Against this background, the adverse influence of school failure may be greater for Hong Kong students (18). In particular, the study of Cheung (40) indicated the inverse relationship between teachers' negative evaluation and youth problem behavior. In academic-oriented schooling, students with poor academic performance might be easily labeled as failures and might engage in delinquent subculture as a way out to social strain. As commented by Cheung (40), students with frustrating school experiences are due to a host of school factors such as difficult curriculum, heavy schoolwork, ineffective teaching, and strong competition among classmates. Encouragement, understanding, and care from teachers are recommended to help students to cope with the tough school reality.

At the individual level, same as prior studies (21-23), the present findings showed that students with better psychosocial competencies were less likely to engage in problem behavior. In particular, compared with other psychosocial correlates, positive youth development qualities and prosocial attributes were the highest protective factors against delinquency. This finding thus echoed the importance of positive youth development programs among adolescents. Through building individual skills and strengthening prosocial connectedness to family, school, and peers, positive youth programs have achieved great success in risk prevention in both local and Western contexts (45). In North America, Catalano et al. (46) found that around 96% of the 25 well-evaluated positive youth development programs reduced problem behavior; whereas in Hong Kong, Shek (23,47) found that positive youth development was negatively correlated with adolescent problem behavior. However, an unexpected finding was found on the positive association of cognitive-behavioral competencies and positive identity with delinquency and problem behavior intention. Perhaps, students who engaged in problem behavior might have "inflated" self-identity and over-estimate their abilities. They might regard their behavior as a rational way to gain popularity and recognition among deviant peers (4). However, when the total scores of positive youth development were used, a negative relationship was still revealed. The present findings suggest that there is a need to look at different aspects of positive youth development and adolescent problem behavior.

Same as both local and Western literature (8,17,19-21), significant gender differences were found in this study. Male students were more likely to engage in problem behavior compared to their female counterparts. In particular, they were more involved in violent activities like assault, gang fighting, and damaging others' properties (19,20). One possible explanation of this finding is the differential gender socialization for boys and girls. While males are socialized to parenting practices that promote physically aggressive behavior, females are socialized to parenting practices that promote caring and closeness (48). However, as commented by Storvoll and Wichstrom (8), "whether or not gender differences were detected was highly dependent on the aspect of conduct problems considered" (p.196). Although boys were more exposed to physical violence, theft, and vandalism (8,19,20), girls were found more likely to consider attempting suicide (19,20). Some studies also indicated that girls engaged in more relational aggression than boys (48). In view of the finding that girls are more likely to engage in covert problem behaviors, parents and school personnel need to be more sensitive to and provide appropriate support to girls under distress. Consistent gender differences found on youth problem behavior have provided insights on gender-specific prevention work.

Although this study has its merit of a large sample from a group of schools in different districts, two limitations must be noted. First, this paper did not examine peer influence on youth delinquency. Numerous Western and local studies indicated that deviant peer influence is one of the strongest predictors of adolescent problem behavior (4,18). In particular, Davis et al. (18) found that peer, family, and school together accounted for 58% of the variance in delinquent behavior of Hong Kong adolescents. More researches should be conducted to take this factor into account. Second, this study only examined the pattern of problem behavior and psychosocial correlates at a particular grade level. To better understand the changing pattern of delinquency and relative influence of psychosocial correlates by age and grade level, a longitudinal study is recommended to trace student development across time. This is what the extension phase of the Project P.A.T.H.S., which is financially supported by the Hong Kong Jockey Club Charities Trust, is attempting to do – to build up a six-year longitudinal database to observe the development of Chinese adolescents in their secondary school years.

In general, this study provides a descriptive profile of delinquency among Hong Kong early adolescents. Despite the general low reported rates of problem behavior, attention should be paid to students' behaviors of cheating, speaking foul language, and drinking alcohol. In view of the predictive power of academic competence, family functioning, and general positive youth development on delinquency, it sheds light on the collaboration of school and family for positive youth development work. It is suggested that school-based positive youth development programs such as the Project P.A.T.H.S. might represent a promising direction for preventing problem behavior by strengthening the psychosocial competencies and family relationships of the participants (23,47,49-52).

ACKNOWLEDGMENTS

This chapter is based upon a paper published in the International Journal on Disability and Human Development (Shek DTL, Ma CMS, Tang CYP. Delinquency and problem behavior intention among early adolescents in Hong Kong. Int J Disabil Hum Dev 2012;11(2):151-8). Permission has been obtained from the publisher to publish this modified version of the paper in this book.

REFERENCES

[1] Hall GS. Adolescence: its psychology and its relation to physiology, anthropology, sociology, sex, crime, religion, and education (Vols. I & II). Englewood Cliffs, NJ: Prentice-Hall; 1904.

[2] Arnett JJ. Adolescent storm and stress, reconsidered. Am Psychol 1999;54:317-26.

[3] Jessor R. Problem-behavior theory, psychosocial development, and adolescent problem drinking. Br J Addict 1987;82:331-42.

[4] Spooner C. Causes and correlates of adolescent drug abuse and implications for treatment. Drug Alcohol Rev 1999;18:453-75.

[5] Barber BK. Family, personality, and adolescent problem behaviors. J Marriage Fam 1992;54:69-79.

[6] Cooper ML, Wood PK, Orcutt HK, Albino AW. Personality and predisposition to engage in risky or problem behaviors during adolescence. J Pers Soc Psychol 2003;84:390-410.

[7] Merikangas KR, Dierker L, Fenton B. Familial factors and substance abuse: implications for prevention. In: Ashery RS, Robertson EB, Kumpfer KL, eds. Drug abuse prevention through family interventions. NIDA Research Monograph no.177. Rockville, MD: National Institute on Drug Abuse, 1998 :12-41.

[8] Storvoll EE, Wichstrom L. Do the risk factors associated with conduct problems in adolescents vary according to gender? J Adolesc 2002;25:183-202.

[9] Joseph Rowntree Foundation. A national survey of problem behaviour and associated risk and protective factors among young people. Joseph Rowntree Foundation 2002. Accessed 2011 Jul 29. URL: http://www.jrf.org.uk/sites/files/jrf/432.pdf

[10] Eccles J, Midgley C, Buchanan CM, Wigfield A, Reuman D, MacIver D. Developmental during adolescents: the impact of stage/environment fit. Am Psychol 1993;48:90-101.

[11] Fishbein M. A theory of reasoned action: some applications and implications. In: Howe H, Page M, eds. Nebraska symposium on motivation. Lincoln, NB: University of Nebraska Press, 1980;27:65-116.

[12] Ajzen I. The theory of planned behavior. Organ Behav Hum Decis Process 1991;50: 179-211.

[13] Rogers RW. Cognitive and physiological processes in fear appeals and attitude change: a revised theory of protection and motivation. In: Cacioppo BL, Petty LL, eds. Social psychophysiology: a sourcebook. London: Guilford, 1983:153-74.

[14] Villarruel AM, Jemmott JB, Jemmott LS, Ronis, DL. Predictors of sexual intercourse and condom use intentions among Spanish-dominant Latino youth: a test of the planned behavior theory. Nurs Res 2004;53(3):172-81.

[15] Buhi E, Goodson P. Predictors of adolescent sexual behavior and intention: a theory-guided systematic review. J Adolesc Health 2007;40:4-21.
[16] Conner M, Sherlock K, Orbell S. Psychosocial determinants of ecstasy use in young people in the UK. Br J Health Psychol 1998;3:295-317.
[17] Drew PY, Watkins D. Sex differences in problem behaviour and the self-concept: an investigation of Hong Kong junior secondary school students. New Horizons in Education 1996;37:11-8.
[18] Davis C, Tang C, Ko J. The impact of peer, family and school on delinquency: a study of at risk Chinese adolescents in Hong Kong. Int Soc Work 2004;47(4):489-502.
[19] Lee A, Tsang CKK. Youth risk behavior in a Chinese population: a territory-wide youth risk behavioral surveillance in Hong Kong. Public Health 2004;118:88-95.
[20] Lee A, Tsang CKK, Lee S, To C. A YRBS survey of youth risk behavior at alternative high schools and mainstream high schools in Hong Kong. J Sch Health 2001:71(9):443-7.
[21] Lam TH, Stewart SM, Ho LM. Prevalence and correlates of smoking and sexual activity among Hong Kong adolescents. J Adolesc Health 2001;29(5):352-8.
[22] Sun RCF, Shek DTL. Life satisfaction, positive youth development and problem behaviour among Chinese adolescents in Hong Kong. Soc Indic Res 2010;95(3):455-74.
[23] Sun RCF, Shek DTL. Positive youth development, life satisfaction and problem behavior among Chinese adolescents in Hong Kong: a replication. Soc Indic Res 2011, in press.
[24] Shek DTL. Family environment and adolescent psychological well-being, school adjustment, and problem behavior: a pioneer study in a Chinese context. J Genet Psychol 1997;158(1):113-28.
[25] Grunbaum JA, Kann L, Kinchen SA, et al. Youth risk behavior surveillance: national alternative high school youth risk behavior survey, United States, 1998. J Sch Health 2000;70(1):5-17.
[26] Eaton DK, Kann L, Kinchen S, et al. Youth risk MMWR Surveill Summ 2010;59(5):1-142.
[27] Lau M, Kan MY. Prevalence and correlates of problem behavior among adolescents in Hong Kong. Asia Pac J Public Health 2010;22(3):354-64.
[28] Hui EKP. Personal concerns and their causes: perceptions of Hong Kong Chinese adolescent students. J Adolesc Health 2000;23:189-203.
[29] Leung PW, Salili F, Baber FM. Common adolescent problems in Hong Kong: their relationship with self esteem, locus of control, intelligence and family environment. Psychologia 1986;29:91-101.
[30] Li SF, Ng RNK. Life stressors and help-seeking behaviour of secondary school students in Kwun Tong: a comprehensive study of students' and their teachers' perception. Hong Kong: Kwun Tong District Committee on Promotion of Mental Health Education, 1992.
[31] Shek DTL. Paternal and maternal influences on the psychological well-being, substance abuse, and delinquency of Chinese adolescents experiencing economic disadvantages. J Clin Psychol 2005;61:219-34.
[32] Shek DTL, Ma CMS. Dimensionality of the Chinese Positive Youth Development Scale: confirmatory factor analyses. Soc Indic Res 2010;98:41-59.
[33] Shek DTL. Assessment of family functioning: the Chinese version of the Family Assessment Device. Res Soc Work Prac 2002;12:502-24.
[34] Shek DTL. Assessment of family functioning Chinese adolescents: the Chinese Family Assessment Instrument. In: Singh NN, Ollen-dick T, Singh AN, eds. International perspectives on child and adolescent mental health. Amsterdam: Elsevier, 2002:297-316.
[35] Siu AMH, Shek DTL. Psychometric properties of the Chinese Family Assessment Instrument in Chinese adolescents in Hong Kong. Adolesc 2005;40:817-30.
[36] Shek DTL. Family functioning and psychological well-being, school adjustment, and substance abuse in Chinese adolescents: are findings based on multiple studies consistent? In: Shohov SP, ed. Advances in psychology research. New York: Nova Science, 2003:163-84.
[37] Shek DTL, Ma CMS. The Chinese Family Assessment Instrument (C-FAI): hierarchical confirmatory factor analyses and factorial invariance. Res Soc Work Pract 2010;20(1):112-23.
[38] Arnett JJ, Jensen LA. Socialization and risk behavior in two countries: Denmark and the United States. Youth Soc 1994;26:3-22.
[39] Hirschi T. Causes of delinquency. Berkeley, CA: University of California, 1969.

[40] Cheung YW. Family, school, peer and media predictors of adolescent deviant behavior in Hong Kong. J Youth Adolesc 1997;26(5):569-96.
[41] Ma HK, Shek DTL, Cheung PC, Lam, COB. Parental, peer and teacher influences on the social behavior of Hong Kong Chinese adolescents. J Genet Psychol 2000;16(1):65-78.
[42] Ho, DYF. Chinese patterns of socialization: a critical review. In: Bond M, ed. The psychology of the Chinese people. Hong Kong: Oxford University Press, 1986:1-37.
[43] Chen X, Dong O, Zhou H. Authoritative and authoritarian parenting practices and social and school performance in Chinese children. Int J Behav Dev 1997;21:855-73.
[44] Lai KW, McBride-Chang C. Suicidal ideation, parenting style, and family climate among Hong Kong adolescents. Int J Psychol 2001;36(2):81-7.
[45] Guerra NG, Bradshaw CP. Linking the prevention of problem behaviors and positive youth development: core competencies for positive youth development and risk prevention. New Dir Child Adolesc Dev 2008;122:1-17.
[46] Catalano RF, Berglund ML, Ryan JAM, Lonczak HS, Hawkins JD. Positive youth development in the United States: research findings on evaluations of positive youth development programs. Ann Am Acad Pol Soc Sci 2004;591:98-124.
[47] Shek DTL, Ma CMS. Impact of the Project P.A.T.H.S. in the junior secondary school years: individual growth curve analyses. ScientificWorldJournal 2011;11:253-66.
[48] Carlo G, Raffaelli M, Laible DJ, Meyer KA. Why are girls less physically aggressive than boys? Personality and parenting mediators of physical aggression. Sex Roles 1999;40:711-29.
[49] Shek DTL, Ng CSM. Early identification of adolescents with greater psychosocial needs: an evaluation of the Project P.A.T.H.S. in Hong Kong. Int J Dis Hum Dev 2010;9:291-9.
[50] Shek DTL, Ng CSM, Tsui PF. Qualitative evaluation of the project P.A.T.H.S.: findings based on focus groups. Int J Dis Hum Dev 2010;9:307-13.
[51] Shek DTL, Yu L. Prevention of adolescent problem behavior: longitudinal impact of the Project P.A.T.H.S. in Hong Kong. ScientificWorldJournal 2011;11:546-67.
[52] Shek DTL, Sun RCF. Secondary data analyses of subjective outcome evaluation findings of the Project P.A.T.H.S. in Hong Kong. ScientificWorldJournal 2010;10:2101-11.

In: Adolescence and Behavior Issues in a Chinese Context ISBN: 978-1-62618-614-9
Editors: DTL Shek, RCF Sun and Joav Merrick

Chapter 7

PERCEPTION OF COUGH MEDICINE AMONG YOUNG SUBSTANCE ABUSERS IN HONG KONG

Daniel T.L. Shek, PhD, FHKPS, BBS, JP[1,2,3,4,5 *]

[1]Department of Applied Social Sciences,
The Hong Kong Polytechnic University, Hong Kong, PRC
[2] Centre for Innovative Programmes for Adolescents and Families,
The Hong Kong Polytechnic University, Hong Kong, PRC
[3]Department of Social Work, East China Normal University,
Shanghai, PRC
[4]Kiang Wu Nursing College of Macau, Macau, PRC
[5]Division of Adolescent Medicine, Department of Pediatrics,
Kentucky Children's Hospital, University of Kentucky College of Medicine,
Lexington, KY, US

ABSTRACT

Although cough medicine abuse is a growing problem in many places, there is no study examining the views of young substance abusers toward cough medicine. The objective of this study was to examine personal constructions of cough medicine abusers via the repertory grid tests (N=11). Several observations are highlighted from the study. First, personal constructions of cough medicine were mixed, including the benefits and harmful effects of its abuse. Second, although the informants perceived cough medicine to be addictive and harmful, they perceived cough medicine to be less addictive and less harmful than did heroin. Third, while the informants construed cough medicine to be similar to ketamine and marijuana, they also perceived cough medicine to possess some characteristics of heroin. Fourth, relative to the construed similarity between heroin and the gateway drugs (cigarette, beer, and liquor), the informants construed cough medicine to be more similar to the gateway drugs. Finally, a higher level of perceived dissimilarity

* Correspondence: Professor Daniel T.L. Shek, PhD, FHKPS, BBS, JP, Chair Professor of Applied Social Sciences, Faculty of Health and Social Sciences, Department of Applied Social Sciences, The Hong Kong Polytechnic University, Room HJ407, Core H, Hunghom, Hong Kong. E-mail: daniel.shek@polyu.edu.hk.

between cough medicine and gateway drugs was related to a higher level of perceived harm of cough medicine abuse.

INTRODUCTION

Adolescent substance abuse is a rising problem in the global contexts. However, while much attention has been spent on the use of cannabis and amphetamine-related drugs in the past few years, less attention has been directed to the abuse of licit drugs that can be bought over the counter (i.e., OTC drugs), such as cough medicine. There are reports on the possible abuse of cough medicine in the United States and Denmark (1,2). According to the press release of the Students for Sensible Drug Policy (3), officials in the United States found that abuse of cough medicine containing dextromethorphan had been intensified among the youth. The findings reported by the Child and Adolescent Workgroup of the National Institute on Drug Abuse in the United States also indicated that the use of cough medicine increased in Grade 10 and Grade 11 students (4). Similar warning was given by the Teen OTC and Prescription Drug Abuse (5).

It was reported that the sale for cough medicine containing opiate constituents ranked highest for non-prescription sales in the United Kingdom (6). According to the BBC Online Network (7), some addicts in the United Kingdom consumed Nurofen Plus, which was made up of ibuprofen and codeine, to get high. Regarding the factors contributing to the abuse of cough medicine, Darboe (8) proposed a theoretical model in which four factors were identified: availability factor, approval factor, ignorance factor, and fear factor. Based on a survey of school personnel, Darboe, Keenan and Richards (9) asserted that "abuse of cough syrup (Robitussin or other brands) has increased over the years and is increasingly perceived as a problem by the community" (p.633).

Cough medicine abuse is also a growing problem in Asia. The prevalence of cough medicine abuse was serious in some Asian countries (10) and codeine was illegally used for abuse purpose in Bangladesh, Malaysia and Myanmar (11). In Malaysia and Myanmar, cough medicine containing codeine was often used in combination with other drugs (10). Besides the illicit use of cannabis and alcohol in Nepal, licit codeine-based medicines had continued to be abused (12). According to a report of Medical Tribune Online (13), the situation in Malaysia was so bad that the Drug Control Authority banned all codeine-based cough preparations starting January 1, 2003. Besides, increased abuse of cough mixture was reported in Japan (14,15) and India (16,17). Mattoo, Basu, Sharma, Balaji and Malhotra (18) studied the socio-demographic and clinical profiles of 46 patients abusing codeine-containing cough syrups (CCS). Findings showed that friends and curiosity were the main reasons for abuse and "the combination of an opioid and a sympathomimetic agent in the CCS may cause a special, distinct euphoric effect" (p.1783).

With specific reference to Hong Kong, several sources of information can give an indication of the severity of the problem. The first source of information is based on the Central Registry of Drug Abuse (19). Generally speaking, abuse of cough medicine has been on the rising trend in the past few years, although there are some fluctuations. Another source of information is from the school surveys regularly conducted by the Narcotics Division (20-24). In a recent school survey, it was found that cough medicine abuse was ranked fourth in the drugs commonly abused by psychotropic drugs taking students (following ketamine, cannabis and ecstasy) with 26.4% of the students abusing the drug (25).

The third source of information is based on the studies conducted or sponsored by the Narcotics Division of the Security Bureau of the Hong Kong Government. For example, in a study of young drug abusers, Narcotics Division (26) showed that heroin, cannabis, and cough medicine were three most commonly abused drugs. Narcotics Division (27) reported that among the 1,110 respondents responding to the question of "Do you know what is the most commonly abused drug in Hong Kong?", 16.8% of the respondents perceived cough medicine to be a drug commonly abused. With reference to "other drugs" perceived by the respondents to be commonly abused in Hong Kong, 48.5% of the respondents perceived cough medicine to be a drug commonly abused by people in Hong Kong. In another study of psychoactive substance abusers of PS33, Lai (28) showed that cough medicine was a major primary drug of abuse among detoxified and non-detoxified subjects. With reference to students' use of a drug within 30 days and knowledge of other drug users, Day and Lee (29) showed that cough medicine was a drug commonly abused by students.

The fourth source of information is based on research conducted by academics and psychiatrists. Based on a retrospective study of 27 patients, Lam, Lee, Shum and Chen (30) showed that the major psychiatric presentations of cough medicine abuse included acute organic brain damage, schizophreniform psychosis and affective episode and remarked "cough mixture misuse has become a focus of concern in Hong Kong since the 1980s" (p.1375). In a study comparing high school students with incarcerated offenders in Hong Kong, Wong, Tang and Schwarzer (31) found that cough medicine abuse was related to attitudes, intentions to try and peer drug use. The final source of information comes from the research conducted by the non-governmental organizations (NGOs). With the intensification of the problem of adolescent substance abuse, many NGOs have conducted researches on adolescent substance abuse that has covered cough medicine abuse. For example, Caritas Aberdeen Outreaching et al (32) showed that among those who had been to rave parties and discos (N=151), 12 respondents (7.9%) had abused cough medicine.

One observation that can be highlighted from the above studies is that studies on attitudes to and beliefs about cough medicine are almost non-existent, although there are some studies on attitudes to substance abuse in general. In a study conducted by the Narcotics Division on public attitude towards substance abuse (27), 76.4% of the respondents agreed that "once people start taking drugs it can be too late" and 96.3% of the respondents agreed that "drugs are dangerous and easily addictive". Another study conducted by the Narcotics Division (26) also showed that 26.2% of the respondents agreed that they could control their heroin taking habit and not get addicted to the drug. Based on qualitative findings, Narcotics Division (33) also reported that psychotropic substances abusers believed that they could control the dosage of drug intake to produce the desired effect without losing control.

Students' attitudes toward substance abuse were also examined in Lau (20). The following findings were reported: 87.4% agreed that "taking heroin is harmful to one's health"; 84.4% agreed that "taking substance like pills, cannabis, cough medicine, solvent thinner is harmful to health"; 81.9% agreed that "taking ecstasy / ketamine is harmful to health"; 84% agreed that "drug abuse destroys your future"; 17.6% agreed that "nowadays, taking pills and cannabis is a hobby, just as smoking"; 15.7% of the respondents agreed that "I can control my heroin taking habit to make heroin taking not addictive"; 19.5% of the respondents agreed that "I can control my habit of taking ecstasy / ketamine to make ecstasy /

ketamine taking not addictive"; 20.7% agreed that "I can control my drug taking habit to make substance abuse not addictive".

In another study conducted by Chiu and Wong (34), attitude and values of children and adolescents toward substance abuse were examined. The researchers examined values about substance abuse via three items: "because adolescents abusing drugs just want to pursue happiness, there is no big deal about this"; "adolescents who want to have fun around should not be fearful about drugs"; "if you don't hurt anybody, there is no harm in taking drugs". The conclusion of the study was that while 67% of the participants held "low" deviant values, 29.1% and 4% had "medium" and "high" deviant values, respectively. However, one limitation of the study is that it is not clear how the different levels of deviant values were operationally defined.

As there is no scientific study on cough medicine abusers' attitudes toward cough medicine, the objective of this study was to examine young substance abusers' personal constructions of cough medicine in relation to different types of drugs and non-drugs via the repertory grid test based on personal construct psychology.

According to Kelly (35), the universe is an ongoing process which can only be understood in terms of construction and re-construction (e.g., from a "safe" drug to "dangerous" drug) through the personal constructs of a person which refer to the world views, interpretations, and deductions about life. Actually, personal constructs are transparent templates, through which the external reality is understood, or categories of thoughts by which an individual construes or interprets his personal world (e.g. 'becoming high' versus 'not becoming high' after consumption). Personal construct psychology has been used in different areas, including psychotherapy, personality assessment, organizational psychology, and education.

The repertory grid test is an assessment method closely related to personal construct psychology that assesses the personal construct system of an individual (36-38). There are three unique features of the repertory grid test. First, the assessment method assesses the individual's subjective worldview from the perspective of the individual (i.e., using the language of the informant). Second, the assessment method can yield data that can be analyzed via quantitative as well as qualitative methods. Finally, the repertory grid test is a very flexible method (e.g., adjusting the number of elements and constructs) that can yield very rich information.

In the Chinese context, Shek and Lam (39) used the repertory grid test to examine the effectiveness of a pioneering drug prevention program in Hong Kong. Group analyses of the grid data of the 30 informants showed that the selves of the participants improved in several areas after joining the program. In sum, the informants psychologically identified themselves (i) more with the "Ideal Self"; (ii) less with "A Drug Addict"; (iii) more with "A Successful Person"; (iv) less with "An Unsuccessful Person". Further qualitative findings showed that there are significant changes in the selves of the informants after joining the program. For example, one informant perceived herself as playful, did not understand oneself, had no future, had no goals, failure, non-persuasive, had no self-control, had no power, and did not listen to others before joining the program. However, the informant perceived herself to have the following characteristics after joining the program: mature, understands herself, thinks about the future, has goals, successful, persuasive, has self-control, has power, and accepts others' views. An examination of the grid data showed that the informant perceived herself to be very close to a drug addict and an unsuccessful person before joining the program.

However, she began to identify herself with the ideal self and a successful person after joining the program.

OUR RESEARCH

In our study, a total of 11 informants were invited to complete the grid on a convenience base. All informants were single males aged between 15 to 24 years. Informed consent was obtained from all participants before the commencement of the study. The following 15 elements were used to elicit the constructs:

Element 1: Heroin
Element 2: Cough medicine
Element 3: Organic solvent
Element 4: Marijuana
Element 5: Tranquilizers
Element 6: "Ice"
Element 7: Ecstasy
Element 8: Cocaine
Element 9: Depressants
Element 10: Ketamine
Element 11: Cigarette
Element 12: Beer
Element 13: Liquor
Element 14: Essence of chicken
Element 15: Chewing gum

For each participant, 10 constructs were elicited via the triadic method. For every triad (i.e., three elements), the participant was asked to construct in which most important way two elements were alike but differed from the third one. After the constructs were elicited, the participant was then asked to rate all the elements on the construct (i.e., along the construct and contrast poles) on a 6-point scale, with 4 to 6 represented the construct pole and 1 to 3 represented the contrast pole. Besides the elicited constructs, there were two supplied constructs (addictive vs. non-addictive and lethal vs. non-lethal). The raw data for each grid (15 elements by 12 constructs) were analyzed by the INGRID 72 program (40-41). In the output of the analysis, there is a section on the distances between pairs of elements. Distances between elements represent the psychological distances between elements, with a minimum value of 0, a mean of 1 and it seldom exceeds the value of 2. Therefore, if the distance between a pair of elements is close to zero, it means that they are seen as similar in the psychological space of the person. On the other hand, if the distance between a pair of elements is close to 2, it means that they are seen to be dissimilar in the psychological space of the informant. Based on the distances between elements, the participants' perceptions of cough medicine in relation to different types of drugs and non-drugs can be revealed. Shek and Lam (39) showed that repertory grid test is a very sensitive method to capture the subjective worldviews of the informants.

WHAT DID WE FIND?

Repertory grid test data can be analyzed by both quantitative and qualitative methods (42). For quantitative data analyses, many computer programs are available (43). For the present study, INGRID 72 was used to analyze the data, the details of which can be seen in Slater (40-41). INGRID 72 generates a wide range of information, including distances between elements in the psychological space of the informant. According to Norris and Makhlouf-Norris (44), distance between two elements can be regarded as the degree of similarity or dissimilarity between two elements and this measure can be regarded as an indicator of a person's degree of identification with an element. Stanley (45) used distances between elements to assess psychological and social alienation in young offenders. Local researchers have also used distances between elements to explore the self-identity systems of drug addicts, mental patients, as well as adolescents after joining a positive youth development program (39, 46-47).

Personal construction of cough medicine by the abusers

The informants' construction of the characteristics of cough medicine is summarized in Table 1. An examination of the findings showed that the related constructs could be categorized into four categories. The first category is on the psychological consequences of abusing cough medicine. All informants construed that cough medicine contributed to changes at the cognitive (e.g., poor memory), affective (e.g., feeling happy) and behavioral (e.g., increase in motor activities) levels. Actually, most of the attributes related to cough medicine were perceived psychological benefits of taking cough medicine. The second category was on the addictive nature of cough medicine, with several informants construed that cough medicine was addictive. The third category was on the harmful effects of cough medicine. The final category was related to other aspects of cough medicine, with some informants construed cough medicine as cheap and accessible. With reference to the supplied constructs, the informants perceived cough medicine to be additive (Mean=4.91, SD=0.94) and harmful (Mean=4.73, SD=1.01). However, analyses using Wilcoxon Test showed that the informants perceived cough medicine to be less addictive (Mean=5.82, SD=0.60 for heroin, $z=-2.16$, $p < .05$) and less harmful (Mean=6.00, SD=0.00 for heroin, $z=2.57$, $p < .02$) than heroin. Two observations can be highlighted with respect to the construed characteristics of cough medicine. First, the constructions were mixed where the informants construed both positive and negative consequences of taking cough medicine. Second, some participants perceived that cough medicine was cheap and easily accessible.

Cough medicine versus other drugs

To what extent cough medicine is perceived to be similar or different from other drugs? An examination of the findings in Table 2 showed that the informants perceived that cough medicine was most similar to ketamine and marijuana and least similar to organic solvent.

Table 1. Personal constructions of cough medicine among the informants

Informant	Personal Construction
1	Easy to get addicted, not easily get fainted after consumption, confused after consumption, drug effect not so strong, no good, will make me addicted, relatively cheap, difficult to get
2	Not good for body, not good thing, harmful to body, expensive, accessible, addictive, has bad influence to body, illegal to consume
3	Sexual urge created by the drug not strong, getting "high" after consumption, sleepy after consumption, drug effect strong, addictive, good feeling after consumption, making oneself relaxed, easy to fall asleep after consumption, relatively expensive, relatively harmful to body
4	Makes one become excited, spirit lifting, can control oneself after consumption, makes one feel relaxed, no need to think much after consumption, feeling less stress after consumption, will not feel unhappy after consumption, addictive
5	Not feeling painful after consumption, not feeling faint after consumption, becomes calm after consumption, feeling comfortable after consumption, feeling confused after consumption, feeling relaxed after consumption, want to move after consumption, knowing what one is doing after consumption, harmful to body, feeling at home after consumption
6	Good feeling after consumption, will paralyze you, unconscious after consumption, getting high, will become more unrestricted after consumption, will not losing control, will become braver, more concentrated in work, mind will not become unclear
7	Comfortable after consumption, will become confused, will become high, enjoyable, will become excited, relatively toxic, not painful after consumption, harmful
8	Addictive, getting high after consumption, spirit lifting, not feeling irritable, cheap, good spirit after consumption, confused mind after consumption, poor memory after consumption, feeling happy after consumption
9	Paralyzed after consumption, concentrated after consumption, feeling good, will make closed ones feel sad, bad for body, forget about worries after consumption, like it, easy to quit, completely conscious
10	Addictive, using more money, will get high after taking, accessible, easily get fainted, will not lose control, will not become dull, anesthetic, will become excited after consumption
11	Addictive, will not get confused after consumption, remains clear-minded after consumption, feeling good after consumption, many young people take it, not hallucinated after consumption, like it, comfortable after consumption, harm is great

Table 2. Mean distances between cough medicine and other drugs

Pair	Mean Distance
Cough Medicine and Heroin	.72
Cough Medicine and Organic Solvent	.84
Cough Medicine and Marijuana	.68
Cough Medicine and Tranquilizers	.76
Cough Medicine and "Ice"	.71
Cough Medicine and Ecstasy	.73
Cough Medicine and Cocaine	.75
Cough Medicine and Depressants	.81
Cough Medicine and Ketamine	.67

Table 3. The completed grid form for Informant No. 7

ELEMENTS	1) Heroin	2) Cough Medicine	3) Organic Solvent	4) Marijuana	5) Tranquilizers	6) Ice	7) Ecstasy	8) Cocaine	9) Depressants	10) Ketamine	11) Cigarettes	12) Beer	13) Liquor	14) Essence of chicken	15) Chewing gum	Construct Pole	Contrast Pole
a.	5	6	3	4	5	5	4	6	5	5	4	4	2	6	4	Comfortable	Uncomfortable
b.	3	6	3	4	4	6	6	5	4	5	1	4	4	1	1	Confused	Not confused
c.	5	6	5	4	5	6	6	6	5	5	2	4	6	1	1	Become high	Not become high
d.	5	6	4	5	5	6	6	6	5	6	3	4	3	1	1	Enjoyable	Not enjoyable
e.	5	6	4	5	5	6	5	6	5	6	3	4	4	1	3	Excited after use	Not excited after use
f.	6	5	6	3	5	6	5	5	5	5	2	4	5	1	1	Toxic	Less toxic
g.	1	1	4	2	1	2	1	1	1	1	1	5	5	1	1	Painful after use	Not painful after use
h.	5	6	3	4	5	5	4	6	5	5	4	4	2	6	4	Comfortable	Uncomfortable
i.	1	1	4	2	1	2	1	1	1	1	1	5	5	1	1	Painful after use	Not painful after use
j.	4	5	1	4	4	1	2	2	2	2	6	5	5	6	6	Harmful	Less harmful
k.	6	3	3	3	2	3	2	4	5	5	1	2	2	1	1	Addictive	Not addictive
l.	6	6	5	4	4	6	6	5	5	5	1	2	3	1	1	Will kill you	Will not kill you

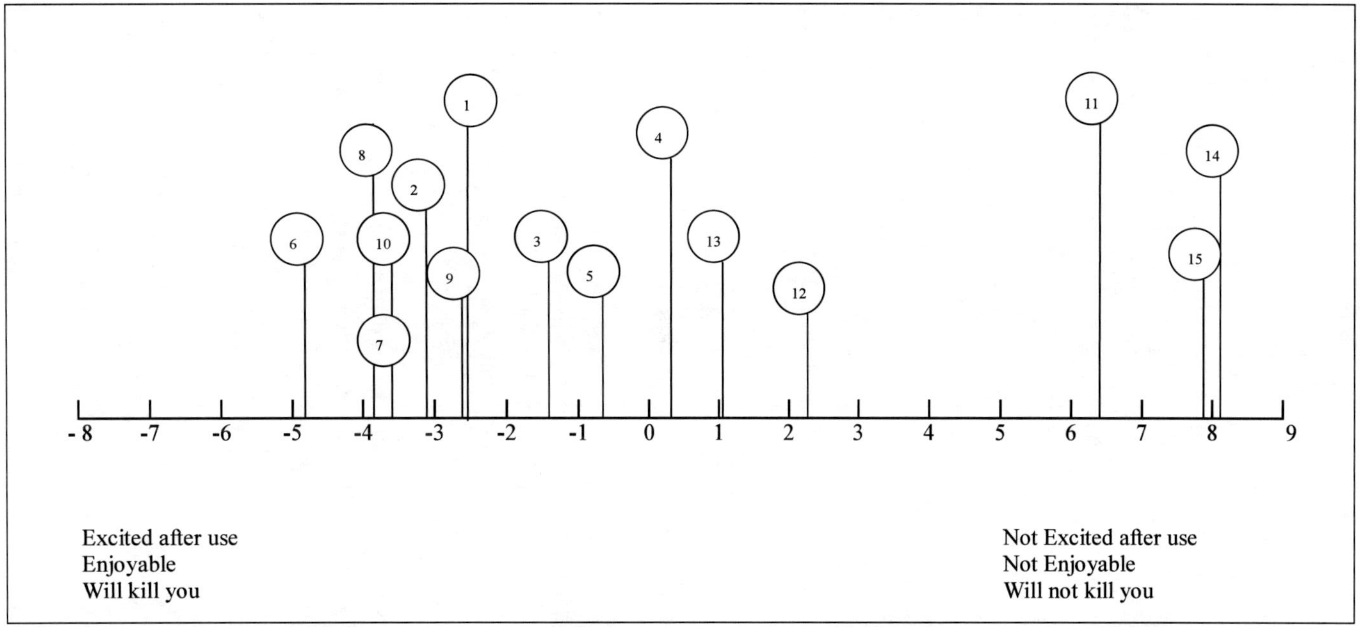

1. Heroin
2.Cough Medicine
3.Organic Solvent
4. Marijuana
5. Tranquilizers
6. "Ice"
7. Ecstasy
8. Cocaine
9. Depressants
10. Ketamine
11. Cigarette
12. Beer
13. Liquor
14. Essence of Chicken
15. Chewing Gum

Figure 1. Representation of cough medicine and other drugs and non-drugs in the psychological space in terms of the first principal component (Informant No. 7).

In other words, the informants appeared to see cough medicine as a kind of “soft drugs”. Nevertheless, results also showed that the informants construed that there was no big difference between cough medicine and heroin. This finding is interesting because it is commonly believed that heroin is very different from cough medicine. In short, the informants construed that cough medicine was similar to soft drugs that also had some characteristics of heroin. An illustration based on Case No. 7 can give some ideas on the informant’s perception of cough medicine and other drugs.

The informant was aged 28 and he had tried heroin, marijuana, tranquilizers, ecstasy, and cough medicine. He began abusing cough medicine at the age of 14. His usual consumption of cough medicine was once every day and he had abused cough medicine for more than once every day in the past three months. On the day of interview, he claimed that he had just consumed a bottle of cough medicine before attending the interview. With reference to Table 3, the informant construed the consumption of cough medicine generating the following characteristics: feeling comfortable (2 times), feeling “wing”, feeling “high”, feeling gratified, feeling excited, relatively more toxic, feeling less painful (2 times), and has greater harm. The informant’s representation of cough medicine and other drugs and non-drugs in his psychological space in terms of the first principal components analysis is presented in Figure 1. In the figure, it is evident that the informant construed the different types of drugs to be relatively the same (that would give “high” and “gratified” feelings but they would kill you) and were very different from the non-drugs.

Cough medicine and other drugs versus non-drugs

Several non-drug elements were utilized in the present study. These included cigarette, beer, liquor, essence of chicken, and chewing gum. Because cigarette, beer, and liquor are commonly regarded as gateway drugs, group analyses were conducted to examine how cough medicine was construed to be similar or different from these gateway drugs. Several observations could be highlighted from the findings:

- Analyses using Wilcoxon Test showed that the mean distance between Element 1 (Heroin) and Element 11 (Cigarette) was significantly longer than the mean distance between Element 2 (Cough Medicine) and Element 11 (Cigarette): $z=-2.22$, $p < .05$. In other words, relative to the construed similarity between heroin and cigarette, the informants construed cough medicine to be more similar to cigarette. The difference is graphically presented in Figure 2.
- Analyses using Wilcoxon Test showed that the mean distance between Element 1 (Heroin) and Element 12 (Beer) was significantly longer than the mean distance between Element 2 (Cough Medicine) and Element 11 (Beer): $z=-2.31$, $p < .05$. In other words, relative to the construed similarity between heroin and beer, the informants construed cough medicine to be more similar to beer. The difference is graphically presented in Figure 3.
- Analyses using Wilcoxon Test showed that the mean distance between Element 1 (Heroin) and Element 13 (Liquor) was significantly longer than the mean distance between Element 2 (Cough Medicine) and Element 13 (Liquor): $z=-2.05$, $p < .05$. In

other words, relative to the construed similarity between heroin and liquor, the informants construed cough medicine to be more similar to liquor. The difference is graphically presented in Figure 4.

An illustration based on Case No. 3 can give some ideas on the informant's construction of cough medicine in relation to the non-drugs. The informant was aged 32 and he had tried heroin, marijuana, tranquilizers, ice, and cough medicine. He began abusing cough medicine at the age of 22 with an usual consumption at 2-6 times every week. He had abused cough medicine 2-6 times each week in the past three months. With reference to Table 4, the informant construed cough medicine had the following characteristics after consumption: creating weak sexual impulse, feeling "high", feeling down, brings quick psychological reaction, addictive, having good, feeling relaxed, easy to sleep, relatively expensive, and has greater harm on the body. The informant's representation of cough medicine and other drugs and non-drugs in his psychological space is presented in Figure 5. In the figure, it is evident that the informant construed cough medicine to be similar to beer (Element 12) and liquor (Element 13).

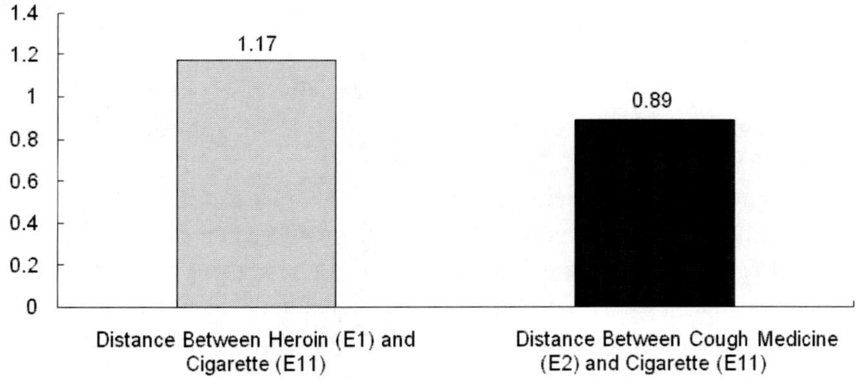

Figure 2. Mean distance between Heroin (E1) and Cigarette (E11) vs. mean distance between Cough Medicine (E2) and Cigarette (E11).

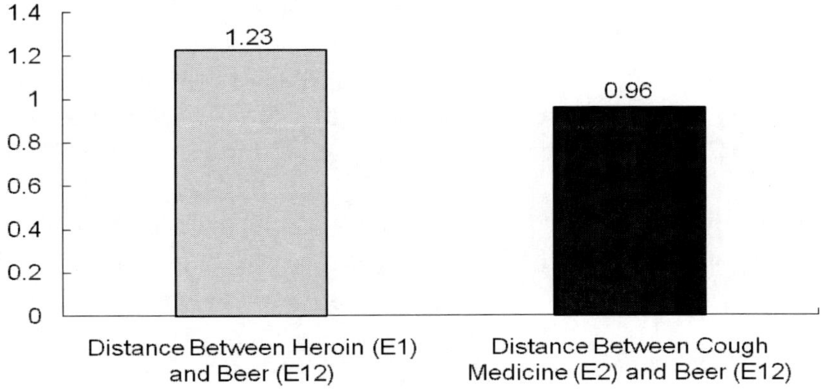

Figure 3. Mean distance between Heroin (E1) and Beer (E12) vs. mean distance between Cough Medicine (E2) and Beer (E12).

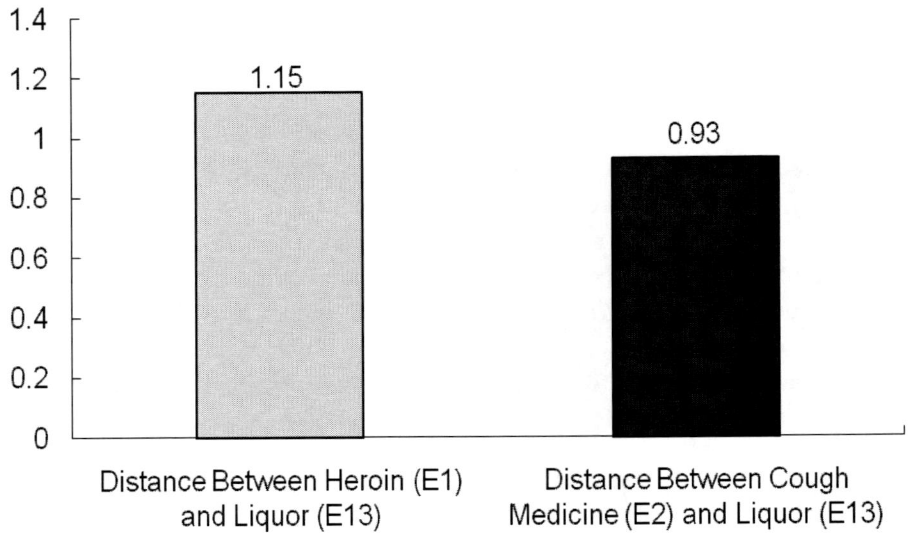

Figure 4. Mean distance between Heroin (E1) and Liquor (E13) vs. mean distance between Cough Medicine (E2) and Liquor (E13).

Another illustration based on Case No. 10 can also give some ideas on the informant's construction of cough medicine in relation to the non-drugs. The informant was aged 34 and he had only abused cough medicine.

He began abusing cough medicine at the age of 31. His usual consumption of cough medicine was 2-6 times each week and he had abused cough medicine once a week in the past three months. With reference to Table 5, the informant perceived that cough medicine had the following characteristics: easily addicted, expensive, feeling "high" after consumption (2 times), easy to get, not feeling dizzy after consumption, lose self-control if taken excessively, not feeling dull after consumption, feeling sedated after consumption, and feeling excited after consumption.

The informant's representation of cough medicine and other drugs and non-drugs in his psychological space is presented in Figure 6. In the figure, it is evident that while the informant construed cough medicine to be similar to beer (Element 12) and liquor (element 13), cough medicine was seen to be different from most of the drugs (except organic solvents).

Pearson correlation analyses showed that a higher level of construed similarity between cough medicine and the gateway drugs was related to a lower level of construed harm of cough medicine ($r=.33$, $p=.33$ for cigarette; $r=.70$, $p < .05$ for beer, and $r=.53$, $p < .10$ for liquor).

In other words, for those who construed that there was high dissimilarity between cough medicine and the gateway drugs, they tended to perceive that cough medicine had greater harm.

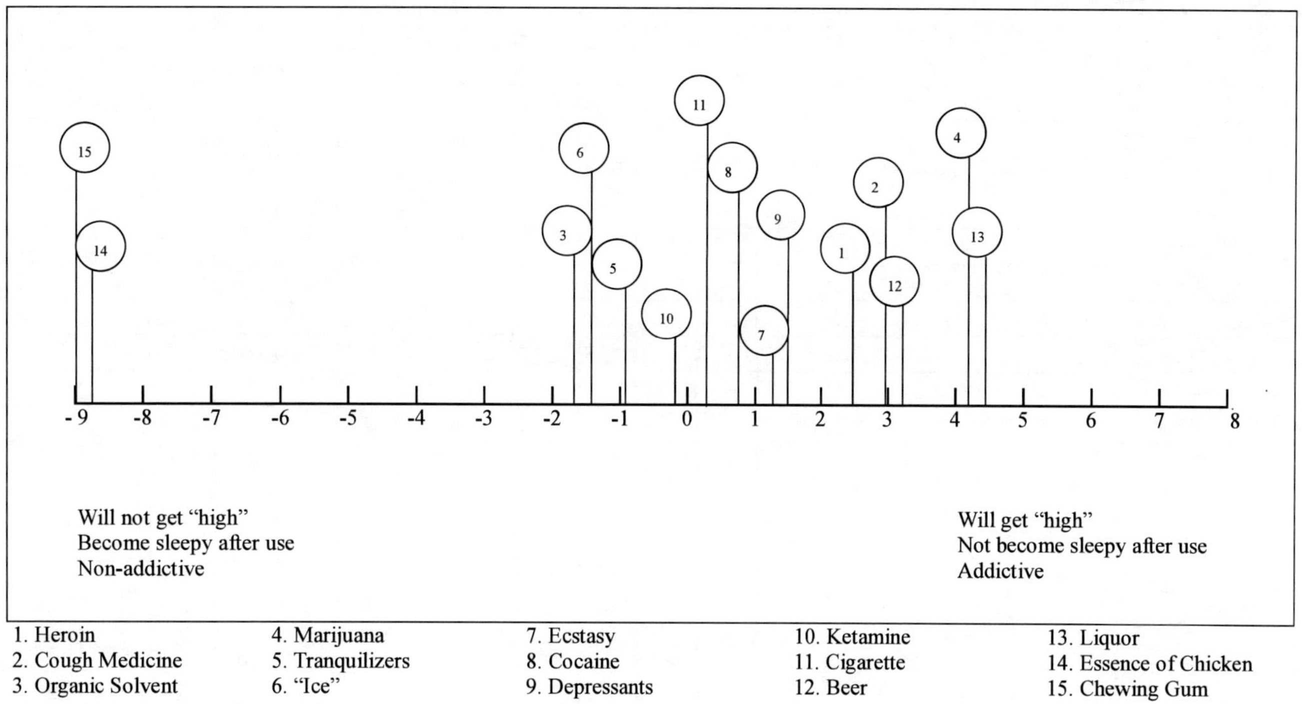

Figure 5. Representation of cough medicine and other drugs and non-drugs in the psychological space in terms of the first principal component (Informant No. 3).

Table 4. The completed grid form for Informant No. 3

ELEMENT	1) Heroin	2) Cough Medicine	3) Organic Solvent	4) Marijuana	5) Tranquilizers	6) Ice	7) Ecstasy	8) Cocaine	9) Depressants	10) Ketamine	11) Cigarettes	12) Beer	13) Liquor	14) Essence of chicken	15) Chewing gum	Construct Pole	Contrast Pole
a.	5	3	1	4	2	6	1	6	2	2	1	4	4	6	1	Strong sexual urge	No strong sexual urge
b.	5	4	1	6	1	1	6	5	4	4	3	5	5	1	1	Getting high	Not getting high
c.	3	5	1	5	4	1	2	3	6	3	3	5	6	1	1	Sleepy	Not Sleepy
d.	5	5	6	5	1	4	3	4	5	4	4	5	5	1	1	Drug effect is strong	Drug effect is weak
e.	6	5	5	6	6	4	6	4	6	4	6	6	4	1	1	Addictive	Non-addictive
f.	4	4	3	6	4	4	4	4	5	4	5	6	4	1	1	Feeling good	Not feeling good
g.	3	6	1	3	3	1	1	3	1	4	4	6	5	1	1	Relaxed	Not relaxed
h.	1	4	1	4	5	1	1	3	1	1	1	5	6	1	1	Easy to sleep	Not easy to sleep
i.	1	3	4	5	6	1	1	1	3	2	5	4	1	1	6	Cheap	Expensive
j.	6	5	6	6	4	6	6	4	4	4	5	3	6	1	1	Harmful to body	Less harmful to body
k.	6	6	4	4	5	5	6	5	6	5	6	5	5	1	2	Addictive	Not addictive
l.	6	4	5	6	4	6	6	5	4	4	3	3	6	1	1	Will kill you	Will not kill you

Table 5. The completed grid form for Informant No. 10

ELEMENTS	1) Heroin	2) Cough Medicine	3) Organic Solvent	4) Marijuana	5) Tranquilizers	6) Ice	7) Ecstasy	8) Cocaine	9) Depressants	10) Ketamine	11) Cigarettes	12) Beer	13) Liquor	14) Essence of chicken	15) Chewing gum	Construct Pole	Contrast Pole
a.	6	4	3	3	5	5	2	6	3	4	2	2	4	1	1	Addictive	Not addictive
b.	5	4	2	6	3	5	4	6	4	4	3	2	5	4	1	Using more money	Not using much money
c.	3	4	4	5	5	4	6	5	6	5	2	4	5	1	1	Getting “high”	Not getting “high”
d.	6	1	1	6	4	6	4	6	4	4	1	1	1	1	1	Not accessible	Accessible
e.	3	4	4	5	5	4	6	5	6	5	2	4	5	1	1	Getting “high”	Not getting “high”
f.	4	3	4	6	5	1	5	4	5	6	3	3	4	1	1	Easy to faint	Not easy to faint
g.	6	4	4	5	4	5	5	4	5	5	3	4	5	1	1	Will lose control	Will not lose control
h.	4	3	4	5	5	3	6	4	6	6	3	4	4	1	1	Become dull	Not become dull
i.	5	4	4	5	5	4	6	5	6	4	2	4	5	1	1	Anesthetic	Non-anesthetic
j.	4	3	5	4	6	2	4	4	4	4	4	4	5	6	6	Not excited	Excited
k.	6	4	3	3	5	5	2	6	3	4	2	2	4	1	1	Addictive	Not addictive
l.	6	3	4	4	4	6	5	5	6	5	3	3	3	1	1	Will kill you	Will not kill you

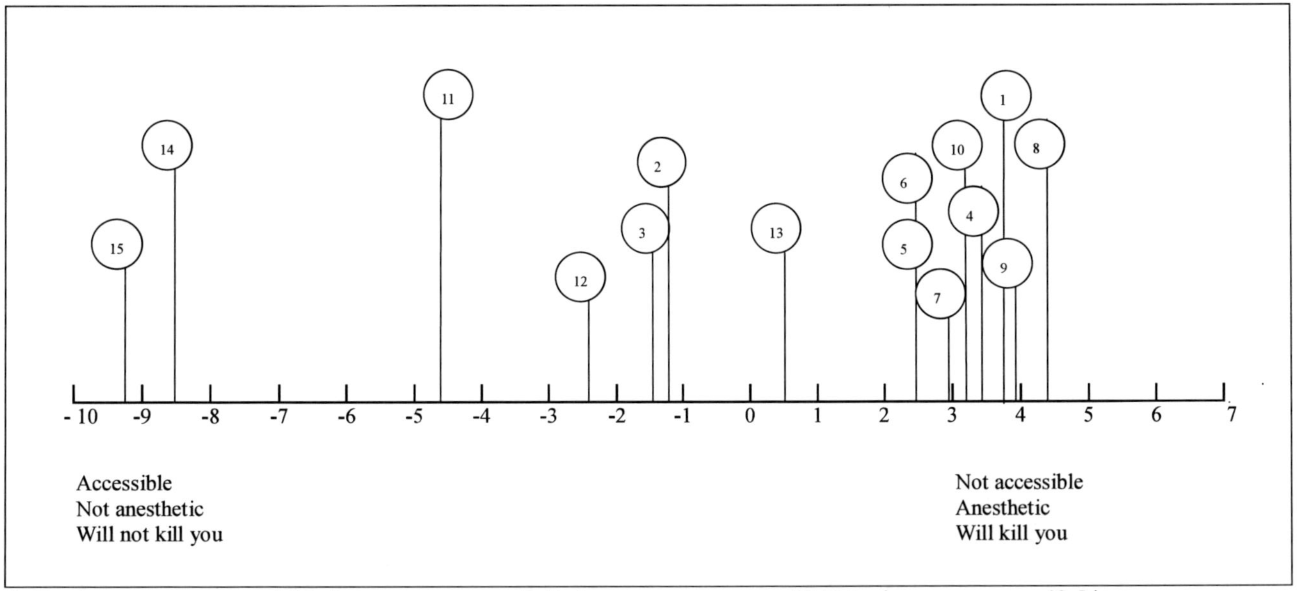

1. Heroin	4. Marijuana	7. Ecstasy	10. Ketamine	13. Liquor
2. Cough Medicine	5. Tranquilizers	8. Cocaine	11. Cigarette	14. Essence of Chicken
3. Organic Solvent	6. “Ice”	9. Depressants	12. Beer	15. Chewing Gum

Figure 6. Representation of cough medicine and other drugs and non-drugs in the psychological space in terms of the first principal component (Informant No. 10).

DISCUSSION

With a few exceptions, there are few studies on cough medicine abuse in the Chinese contexts. Shek and Lam (48) examined beliefs about cough medicine abuse among Chinese young people using the Beliefs about Cough Medicine Abuse Scale (BACMAS), with a total of 225 Chinese young people (160 cough medicine abusers and 65 non-cough medicine abusers) participated in the study. Results showed that the scale was internally consistent. The scale was able to differentiate those who abused and did not abuse cough medicine and a higher level of BACMAS scores was related to higher levels of endorsement of cough medicine abuse and severity of consumption, thus providing support for the concurrent and construct validities of the scale. Regarding attitudes to cough medicine abuse, although the respondents abusing cough medicine generally did not perceive any benefits of abusing cough medicine and they recognized the harmful effects of cough medicine abuse, roughly three-tenth of the respondents believed that cough medicine was not addictive and more than half of them believed that there was no harm to get along with friends abusing cough medicine.

Besides, qualitative data on the views of different stakeholders on cough medicine abuse have been reported. Lam and Shek (49) conducted focus groups based on young cough medicine abusers (N=8), parents of cough medicine abusers (N=5), and social workers (N=6). Several observations were revealed from the qualitative findings. First, all the research participants shared a view that their first use of cough medicine was under the influence of peers and they remarked that they had no problems at all to obtain legally controlled cough medicine from pharmacies. Although there were no obvious discomforts at the initial stage, the participants reported observed harmful effects in the physical, psychological, interpersonal and family domains after prolonged cough medicine use. Second, social factors (mainly peer influence), personal factors (avoidance), family factors (poor family relationship or unhappy family incidents), availability (ease of access), and ignorance (unawareness of the harmful consequences and wrong beliefs) were identified to be the reasons for cough medicine abuse. In particular, family members were generally insensitive to the issue of cough medicine abuse. Emotional and financial problems were major difficulties encountered by the families concerned. Third, there were personal (dependency and wrong beliefs), environmental (accessibility of cough medicine and ignorance of service), and system barriers (loose legal control and stigmatization) to help seeking. Personal factors (self-awareness and insight) and support systems (family and service support) were identified to be the factors facilitating help seeking. Finally, the stakeholders and service providers recommended that there was a need for holistic treatment orientation, collaboration among helping professions, and reaching out. It was also recommended that the Government should be more proactive in community education and stricter law enforcement, and separate hospital arrangements should be made to avoid stigmatization. Although the focus group findings are very revealing, the findings are more related to social construction of cough medicine abuse in the focus groups instead of personal construction of cough medicine abuse.

Against this background, the present study was conducted to understand personal constructions of cough medicine and a personal construct theory was adopted to examine the issue concerned. There are several conclusions of the study. First, personal constructions of cough medicine were mixed and the observation was in line with the findings reported by Shek and Lam (48) and Lam and Shek(49). Practically, it is important to further understand why abusers continue to abuse cough medicine despite their realization of its harmful effect. In addition, it is also important to consider how the construed benefits of cough medicine abuse can be minimized whereas the construed harms can be translated into motivation to quit the drug. Second, regarding the addictive nature of cough medicine, although the informants perceived cough medicine to be additive and harmful, they perceived cough medicine to be less addictive and less harmful than heroin. The finding suggests that the distinction between "hard" and "soft" drugs is still in the minds of the abusers. Third, concerning cough medicine versus other drugs, while the informants construed cough medicine to be similar to Kketamine and marijuana, they also perceived cough medicine to possess some characteristics of heroin. Because cough medicine abusers tend to construe cough medicine as similar to soft drugs, more preventive education and publicity work should be done. While there are anti-heroin and anti-psychotropic substances (such as ecstasy and ketamine) initiatives, there are comparatively fewer anti-cough medicine abuse preventive and publicity attempts, such as APIs and posters.

Fourth, regarding cough medicine and drugs versus other drugs, relative to the construed similarity between heroin and the gateway drugs (cigarette, beer, and liquor), the informants construed cough medicine to be more similar to the gateway drugs. Again, the theme of relatively "milder" harm of cough medicine abuse in comparison with heroin can be seen from the findings. The finding suggests that the abusers might be psychologically less conscious of the unique addictive and harmful effects of cough medicine. More efforts to reduce the "blurred" nature of cough medicine are needed. Fifth, for those who construed that there was high dissimilarity between cough medicine and the gateway drugs, they tended to perceive that cough medicine had greater harm. The finding suggests that there is a need to change the personal constructions of cough medicine abusers. Sixth, consistent with the spirit of personal construct psychology, the present findings suggest that there is a need for helping professionals to thoroughly understand the beliefs and personal construct systems of the abusers of cough medicine. Therapeutically speaking, how to change the personal construction and beliefs about cough medicine of the abusers is an important area for intervention. Finally, the present findings underscore the usefulness of using the repertory grid technique in understanding the subjective worlds of the abusers regarding different types of drugs, including their perceived benefits and harms.

In conjunction to the findings of the present study, several recommendations regarding prevention of cough medicine abuse are proposed. First, as the cough medicine abusers are not fully aware of the addictive nature of cough medicine, there is a need to raise public awareness of the harmful effects of cough medicine via preventive education and publicity initiatives as follows: (a) public, school-based, and family-based preventive education should be carried out, particularly in families with young adolescents; (b) young people should be helped to develop non-permissive and proper beliefs about cough medicine abuse; (c) in view of the relatively lack of preventive education and publicity materials on anti-cough medicine abuse (e.g., posters and APIs), the Government should review the existing anti-cough medicine initiatives and develop timely measures.

Besides, young substance abusers should understand the negative impact of cough medicine abuse. Some researchers have studied the perceived effects of abusing cough medicine. Based on a group of Indian abusers, Mattoo et al. (18) found the following reported effects of taking cough medicine: feeling alert, becoming more active, feeling cheerful, becoming over-talkative, and feeling drowsy. Based on the data collected via focus group discussion, Sung (50) found that cough medicine abusers perceived the following benefits of taking cough medicine: enhancement of concentration on routine jobs, ability to relax and enhancement of energy and excitement. There are other studies showing that abuse of cough medicine produces psychotic states. Krenzelok (51) reported that intake of a large amount of cough syrup might produce phencyclidine (PCP) like effect, hyperactivity as well as hallucination. Mendez (52) suggested that sympathomimetic amines in cough medicine could lead to manic states. With specific reference to dextromethorphan, which is a common ingredient in cough medicine, Fisher (53) commented that if taken in large quantity, dextromethorphan would produce PCP like effect. Price and Liebel (54) reported a case of dextromethorphan-induced psychosis and concluded that "clinicians should be vigilant in treating cases that suggest dextromethorphan abuse" (p.304). Polles and Griffith (55) reported two cases showing that dextromethorphan could cause secondary mania. Bostwick (56) also summarized "the take-home message is that OTC preparations are a potential psychoactive polypharmacy in a bottle and that should be used with caution in patients with predisposition to affective illness by family or personal history" (p.572). In a recent study of cough medicine abuse in Hong Kong, Au et al (57) examined four cases of young men with cough mixture abuse and severe folate deficiency. The four cases presented at least two of following symptoms: difficulty in walking, dizziness, lower limb weakness, numbness in all limbs, axonal degeneration, and dental caries , with the last two symptoms found in most cases.

In addition to preventive drug education and understanding of the nature of cough medicine abuse, promotion of psychosocial competence is also important. As the present findings showed that cough medicine abusers held contradictory beliefs about cough medicine, strengthening their cognitive competence is indispensable. In particular, young people should be helped to understand the role of peers in cough medicine abuse (i.e., social competence). Resistance skills (i.e., behavioral competence) and healthy network building (i.e., bonding) should be emphasized. Besides, strategies that can enhance the coping abilities (i.e., resilience) and reduce the curiosity of young people about drugs should be devised. Young people should be helped to understand the role of family factors in cough medicine abuse and they should learn how to deal with negative emotions about their families (i.e., emotional competencies). In the West, many programs have been developed to promote the psychosocial competencies of young people to stay away from drugs. Nevertheless, while there are successful programs to reduce substance abuse in young people in the West, related effective programs are almost non-existent in the Chinese contexts (58). One notable exception is the Project P.A.T.H.S. in Hong Kong. There are evaluation findings showing that the program was able to promote positive youth development, reduce substance abuse, and delinquency of participants (59-63). It is suggested that there is a need to further promote the program and increase the sustainability of the program in the long run.

There are several contributions of the present research project. First, because no systematic study of cough medicine abuse has been carried out in different Chinese and global contexts, this is a groundbreaking attempt and the present findings contribute to the limited literature. Second, the present study provides additional evidence suggesting that substance abuse among young people is a multi-dimensional problem involving different psychosocial factors. Third, the present study underscores the importance of triangulation in the understanding of cough medicine abuse. Fourth, the present study demonstrates the importance of understanding the psychological worlds of cough medicine abusers. Finally, the scale assessing beliefs about cough medicine abuse is invaluable to drug prevention workers in different Chinese contexts.

Nevertheless, there are also several limitations of the present study. First, because of the cross-sectional design of this research, we need to further investigate the causal processes involved in cough medicine abuse among young people via longitudinal studies. Second, a purposive sample design was adopted in this study. While this design is commonly used in research on drug abuse, its limitations, particularly with respect to the generalizability of the findings, should be duly acknowledged. Third, the sample size of the present study is relatively small, only 11 informants were recruited, which will also affect the generalization of findings. However, this sample size is considered reasonable in qualitative study. Third, if resources permit, participants randomly drawn should be recruited to participate in the repertory grid tests. In particular, a wider range of cough medicine abusers and their parents as well as social workers should be recruited to participate in the related studies. Despite these limitations, this study has provided the most updated information to enrich our understanding of cough medicine abuse among young people in Hong Kong. The policy and service implications of the present findings deserve the attention of young people, parents, teachers, helping professionals, policy makers, and the general public.

REFERENCES

[1] Jensen S, Hansen AC. Abuse of codeine separated from over-the-counter drugs containing acetylsalicylic acid and codeine. Int J Legal Med 1993;105:279-81.

[2] Jinks KJ, Raschko RR. A profile of alcohol and prescription drug abuse in high risk community based elderly population. Drug Inform Clin Pract 1990;24:971-5.

[3] Students for Sensible Drug Policy. Cold medicine abuse spreading among youths: Officials finds 2004. Accessed 2012 Sep 15. URL: http://www.mapinc.org/

[4] National Institute on Drug Abuse. High school and youth trends. Washington, DC: National Institute Drug Abuse, 2011.

[5] Teen OTC and Prescription Drug Abuse. Dextromethorphan. Accessed 2012 Sep 15. URL: http://www.teenoverthecounterdrugabuse.com/

[6] Anonymous. Cough medicines (editorial). Drug Ther Bull 1985;22:85-7.

[7] BBC Online Network. Health pharmacist's painkiller warning. Accessed 2012 Sep 15. URL: http://news.bbc.co.uk.

[8] Darboe MN. Abuse of dextromethorphan-based cough syrup as a substitute for licit and illicit drugs: a theoretical framework. Adolescence 1996;21:239-45.

[9] Darboe MN, Keenan GR, Richards TK. The abuse of dextromethorphan-based cough syrup: a pilot study of the community of Waynesboro, Pennsylvania. Adolescence 1996;31:633-44.

[10] United Nations Office on Drugs and Crime, United Nations. Fact sheets: drug abuse trends in East Asia. Accessed 2012 Sep 15. URL:http://www.unodc.org/

[11] United Nations Office on Drugs and Crime, United Nations. Regional Centre for East Asia and the Pacific. Fact sheets: opium and derivatives. Accessed 2012 Sep 15. URL: http://www.unodc.org/

[12] Bureau for International Narcotics and Law Enforcement Affairs. International Narcotics Control Strategy Report: 2002. Accessed 2012 Sep 15. URL: http://www.state.gov

[13] Medical Tribune Online, Codeine cough mixtures banned from next year. Accessed 2012 Sep 15. URL: http://www.medicaltribune.com

[14] Ishigooka J, Yoshida Y, Murasaki M. Abuse of "BRO NO": A Japanese OTC cough suppressant solution containing methylephedrine, codeine, caffeine and chlorpheniramine. Prog Neuro-Psychoph 1991;15:513-21.

[15] Suzuki T, Masukawa Y, Misawa M. Drug interactions in the reinforcing effects of over-the-counter cough syrups. Psychopharmacology 1990;102:438-42.
[16] Borde M, Nizamie SH. Dependence on a common syrup. Lancet 1988;1:760-1.
[17] Wairagkar NS, Das J, Kumar S. Codeine containing cough syrup addiction in Assam and Nagaland. Indian J Psychiatry 1994;36:129-32.
[18] Mattoo SK, Basu D, Sharma A, Balaji M, Malhotra A. Abuse of codeine-containing cough syrups: a report from India. Addiction 1997;92:1783-7.
[19] Narcotics Division. Central Registry of Drug Abuse (Fifty-eighth Report). Hong Kong: Narcotics Division, Government of the Hong Kong Special Administrative Region, 2010.
[20] Lau JTF. The 2000 survey of drug use among students. Hong Kong: Narcotics Division, Government of Hong Kong, 2002.
[21] Narcotics Division. 1990 survey on the non-medical use of psychotropic substances among students of secondary schools and technical institutes. Hong Kong: Narcotics Division, Government of Hong Kong, 1991.
[22] Narcotics Division. 1992 survey on drug use among students of secondary schools and technical institutes. Hong Kong: Narcotics Division, Government of Hong Kong, 1993.
[23] Narcotics Division. 1996 survey on drug use among students of secondary schools and technical institutes. Hong Kong: Narcotics Division, Government of Hong Kong, 1997.
[24] Narcotics Division. Central Registry of Drug Abuse (Fifty-ninth Report). Hong Kong: Narcotics Division, Government of Hong Kong, 2010.
[25] Narcotics Division. The 2008/09 survey of drug use among students. Hong Kong: Narcotics Division, Government of Hong Kong, 2010.
[26] Narcotics Division. Report on survey of young drug abusers. Hong Kong: Narcotics Division, Security Bureau, Government of Hong Kong, 1994.
[27] Narcotics Division. 1994 Survey to assess public awareness of anti-drug activities. Hong Kong: Narcotics Division, Government of Hong Kong, 1994.
[28] Lai B. A retrospective and a prospective study of psychoactive substance abusers of PS33. Hong Kong: Narcotics Division, Government Secretariat, Government of Hong Kong, 1997.
[29] Day J, Lee C. An evaluation of talks given by the Narcotics Division, Hong Kong Government Secretariat, to students in secondary schools, for prevention of drug abuse. Hong Kong: Drug Addiction Research Unit, Social Sciences Research Center, University of Hong Kong, 1996.
[30] Lam LCW, Lee D, Shum PPS, Chen CN. Cough mixture abuse in Hong Kong. An emergent psychiatric problem? Addiction 1996;91:1375-8.
[31] Wong CSY, Tang CSK, Schwarzer R. Psychosocial correlates of substance use: comparing high school students and incarcerated offenders in Hong Kong. J Drug Educ 1996;27:147-72.
[32] Caritas Aberdeen Outreaching Team. Substance abuse among young people in discos. Hong Kong: Caritas, 2000.
[33] Narcotics Division. Report of the task force on psychotropic substances abuse. Hong Kong: Narcotics Division, Security Bureau, Government of Hong Kong, 2002.
[34] Chiu S, Wong V. A research study on substance abuse among young people in Yuen Long. Hong Kong: Yuen Long District Fight Crime Committee, 2002.
[35] Kelly G. The psychology of personal constructs (Vol 1-2). New York: Norton, 1955.
[36] Fransella F. Repertory Grid Technique. In: Fransella F, ed. Personality: theory, measurement and research. London: Methuen, 1981:166-77.
[37] Fransella F, Bannister D. A manual for repertory grid technique. London: Academic Press, 1977.
[38] Viney LL. Should we use personal construct therapy? A paradigm for outcomes evaluation. Psychotherapy 1998;35:366-80.
[39] Shek DTL, Lam CW. Evaluation of a preventive drug education program in Hong Kong using the repertory grid test. Int Public Health J, in press.
[40] Slater P, ed. The measurement of interpersonal space by grid technique (Vol 1). New York: Wiley, 1976.
[41] Slater P, ed. The measurement of interpersonal space by grid technique (Vol 2). New York: Wiley, 1977.

[42] Bannister D. The rationale and clinical relevance of repertory grid technique. Br J Psychiatry 1965;111:977-82.

[43] Shaw MLG. Recent advances in personal construct technology. London: Academic Press, 1981.

[44] Norris H, Makhlouf-Norris F. The measurement of self-identity. In: Slater P, ed. Explorations of intrapersonal space. New York: Wiley, 1976:79-82.

[45] Stanley B. Alienation in young offenders. In: Beail N, ed. Repertory grid technique and personal constructs: applications in clinical and educational settings. London: Croom Helm, 1985:47-60.

[46] Luk AL, Shek DTL. Perceived personal changes in Chinese ex-mental patients attending a holistic psychiatric rehabilitation program. Soc Behav Personal 2006;34(8):939-54.

[47] Shek DTL. Evaluation of a positive youth development program based on the repertory grid test. Sci World J, Advance online publication. doi: 10.1100/2012/372752.

[48] Shek DTL, Lam CM. Beliefs about cough medicine abuse among Chinese young people in Hong Kong. Soc Behav Personal 2008;36(1): 135-44.

[49] Lam CM, Shek DTL. A qualitative study of cough medicine abuse among Chinese young people in Hong Kong. J Subst Use 2006;11(4):233-44.

[50] Sung E. A focus group study on psychotropic substance abuse. Hong Kong: Narcotics Division, Security Bureau, Government of Hong Kong, 2001.

[51] Krenzelok EP. Non-prescription cough medicine abuse. Clin Toxicol Forum 1990;2:5.

[52] Mendez MF. Mania self-induced with cough syrup. J Clin Psychiatr 1992;53:173-4.

[53] Fisher JD. Dextromethorphan. Clin Toxicol Rev 1991;13:1-2.

[54] Price LH, Liebel J. Dextromethorphan-induced psychosis. Am J Psychiatr 2000;157:304.

[55] Polles A, Griffith JL. Dextromethorphan-induced mania. Psychosomatics 1996;37(1):71-4.

[56] Bostwick JM. Dextromethorphan-induced manic symptoms in a bipolar patient on lithium. Psychosomatics 1996;37:571-2.

[57] Au WY, Tsang J, Cheng TS, Chow WS, Woo YC, Ma SK, Tam S. Cough mixture abuse as a novel cause of megaloblastic anaemia and peripheral neuropathy. Br J Haematol 2003;123:954-9.

[58] Shek DTL, Yu L. A review of validated youth prevention and positive youth development programs in Asia. Int J Adolesc Med Health 2011;23(4):317-24.

[59] Shek DTL, Sun RCF. Subjective outcome evaluation based on secondary data analyses: the Project P.A.T.H.S. in Hong Kong. Sci World J 2010;10:224-37.

[60] Shek DTL, Ng CSM, Tsui PF. Qualitative evaluation of the Project P.A.T.H.S.: findings based on focus groups. Int J Disabil Hum Dev 2010;9:307-13.

[61] Shek DTL. Using students' weekly diaries to evaluate positive youth development programs: are findings based on multiple studies consistent? Soc Indic Res 2010;95(3):475-87.

[62] Shek DTL. Quantitative evaluation of the training program of the Project P.A.T.H.S. in Hong Kong. Int J Adolesc Med Health 2010;21(3):425-35.

[63] Shek DTL, Sun RCF. Secondary data analyses of subjective outcome evaluation findings of the Project P.A.T.H.S. in Hong Kong. Sci World J 2010;10:2101-11.

In: Adolescence and Behavior Issues in a Chinese Context ISBN: 978-1-62618-614-9
Editors: DTL Shek, RCF Sun and Joav Merrick

Chapter 8

SELF-HARM AND SUICIDAL BEHAVIORS IN HONG KONG ADOLESCENTS

Daniel TL Shek, PhD, FHKPS, BBS, JP[1-5] * ***and Lu Yu, PhD***[1]

[1]Department of Applied Social Sciences,
The Hong Kong Polytechnic University, Hong Kong, PRC
[2]Public Policy Research Institute,
The Hong Kong Polytechnic University, Hong Kong, PRC
[3]Department of Social Work, East China Normal University, Shanghai, PRC
[4]Kiang Wu Nursing College of Macau, Macau, PRC
[5]Division of Adolescent Medicine, Department of Pediatrics,
Kentucky Children's Hospital, University of Kentucky College of Medicine,
Lexington, KY, US

ABSTRACT

In this chapter we examine the prevalence and psychosocial correlates of adolescent deliberate self-harm (DSH) and suicidal behavior in a representative sample of 3,328 secondary school students in Hong Kong. With reference to the previous year, 32.7% of the students reported at least one form of DSH; 13.7% of the respondents had suicide thoughts; 4.9% devised specific suicidal plans, and 4.7% had actually attempted suicide. Adolescent girls had significantly higher rates of DSH and suicidal behavior than did adolescent boys. Having re-married parents were related to an increased likelihood of DSH and suicide. While high levels of family functioning, overall positive youth development, and academic and school performance predicted low rates of DSH and suicidal behavior, cognitive and behavioral competence was unexpectedly found to be positively associated with DSH and suicidal behavior. Theoretical and practical implications of the findings are discussed.

* Correspondence: Professor Daniel T.L. Shek, PhD, FHKPS, BBS, JP, Chair Professor of Applied Social Sciences, Faculty of Health and Social Sciences, Department of Applied Social Sciences, The Hong Kong Polytechnic University, Room HJ407, Core H, Hung Hom, Hong Kong. E-mail: daniel.shek@polyu.edu.hk.

INTRODUCTION

Deliberate self-harm (DSH) and suicidal behaviors among adolescents represent major public health problems because they often lead to serious detrimental outcomes. Proximally, DSH and suicide bring physical harm (and even death) to the individual. Distally, DSH and suicidal behavior are related to a wide range of psychopathology, problem behaviors, and poor overall functioning. Although DSH and suicidal behaviors are closely associated, they are qualitatively different (1). DSH is defined as the intentional injury of one's own body tissue without apparent suicidal intent, while suicidal behavior refers to the act of deliberately or intentionally taking one's own life (2,3). Empirical studies conducted in the West have accumulated growing evidence on the rates and correlates of adolescent DSH and suicidal behaviors. In contrast, scientific information about the two phenomena among youth in different Chinese communities is sparse. Against the above background, the present study attempted to examine the prevalence and associated psychosocial factors of deliberate self-harm and suicidal behaviors in Chinese adolescents based on a large sample of secondary school students in Hong Kong.

In the past two decades, researchers have found that DSH has become more and more prevalent in adolescents, although the reported rates of DSH vary across countries. Using anonymous self-report questionnaires, Hawton et al. reported that 6-7% of the surveyed 15-year-old students in England showed at least one episode of DSH during the previous 12 months (4). In the United States, lifetime prevalence of DSH generally ranged from 12% to 37.2% in secondary school students (5-7) and 12% to 20% in late adolescent and young adult populations (8,9). High rates of DSH have also been found in other Western countries. A prevalence rate of 24% was reported among young female adults in Italy (10), whereas a lifetime prevalence rate of 21.4% was found among 839 students in Turkey (11). While DSH may occur at all age, research findings showed that adolescents and young adults are at a higher risk (12). Thus, there is a consensus that adolescence is a risky period in which DSH may occur.

As one of the leading causes of death in adolescents, suicide has always been a subject of continuing research across the world. Specifically, suicidal behavior can be viewed as existing along a continuum from thinking about ending one's life (suicide ideation or thoughts), developing a plan (suicide plan), non-fatal suicidal behavior (suicide attempt), to ending one's life (suicide) (13). In recent years, although the rate of suicide directly resulting in adolescent death (fatal suicidal behaviors) decreases modestly, the prevalence of suicide ideation and suicide attempt (non-fatal suicidal behavior) has been found to be alarmingly high among youth. Based on a large sample of school students in Switzerland, researchers reported that about 26% of the 15 to 20 years old adolescents had suicidal thoughts, 15% had suicidal plans and 3% had suicide attempts (14). In a systematic review of 128 studies, Evans, Hawton, Rodham, and Deeks revealed that on average 9.7% of adolescents reported that they had attempted suicide at some point in their life and that an additional 29.9% of adolescents reported having suicidal thoughts at some point in their lives (15).

Although there are plenty of research-based data on the prevalence of DSH and suicidal behaviors in adolescents from Western countries, particularly the United States, such information is very limited from Asian countries including different Chinese communities. Existing research findings regarding the rates of DSH and suicidal behaviors in Chinese adolescents are equivocal because of the lack of systematic studies and numerous methodological variations, such as utilization of different assessment measures and procedures. For example, based on parent-reported questionnaires, Liu, Sun and Yang found that 3.2% of a community sample of Chinese adolescents had deliberately harmed themselves (16), while a recent study using self-reported questionnaire showed that the prevalence rate of DSH was 15.5% among 2,013 Chinese students aged between 10 to 24 years (17).

With reference to suicide, different prevalence findings were also reported. Liu investigated suicidal behaviors among 1,362 adolescents (mean age = 14.6 years) and found that 19.3% of the sample reported having suicidal ideation and 10.5% having suicide attempts in the past 6 months (18). With a population-based sample, Pan, Zhang, and Shi (19) reported a similar rate of 18.6% of suicidal ideation in 23,976 students aged 12 to 19 years. Yet, Tang et al.'s study showed apparently lower rates: suicidal ideation and suicidal attempts were reported by 8.8% and 3.5% of the participated Chinese adolescents (17). In Hong Kong, 26.8% of a community sample of adolescents reported having ever thought about suicide in their life and 4.5% had suicidal ideation in the past 12 months; among the participants, 2.3% had made a suicide plan in the past year and nearly all of them actually attempted suicide (20). Clearly, the existing mixed findings cannot provide an accurate picture of the situation of DSH and suicidal behavior in Chinese adolescents. As such, there is a great need for systematically examining the two problem behaviors with methodologically sound empirical research.

To effectively prevent DSH and suicidal behaviors, numerous studies have been conducted to identify risk and protective factors for adolescents at different levels. At the individual level, gender was found to be a predictor of DSH. Adolescent girls had significantly higher self-harm rates than did adolescent boys (4,21-23) and patients who utilized medical treatment for self-harm were more often females (24,25). Results regarding gender difference in suicide varied across studies and different suicide-related behaviors. In the United States, research findings have shown that males are four times as likely to kill themselves and females are three to nine times as likely to have attempted suicide (26). Several researchers suggest that adolescent males are prone to use more aggressive suicide methods which increase the likelihood of death (27). In Hong Kong, Chan et al. reported that females had significantly higher rates of lifetime suicide ideation than did males (28). However, it was also showed that there was no significant gender difference in suicide plans and suicide attempts in the past 12 months.

At the family level, a number of studies suggest that different family factors are related to adolescent DSH and suicidal behaviors. First, most findings showed that low family economic status was associated with higher rates of both self-harm and suicidal behaviors among adolescents. For example, several researchers reported that low household income was significantly related to suicidal thoughts among Chinese adolescents (28,29). However, there are also reports suggesting no significant relationship between family financial problem and adolescent self-harm behaviors (30). Second, there has been a link between parental marriage status and adolescent self-harm and suicide-related behaviors. In a longitudinal study, not living in a family with two biological parents at age 12 significantly predicted DSH three years later (31). Researchers also found that divorce of parents can potentially trigger suicidal thoughts in young people (32). Third, severe family dysfunctioning has been found to be a major factor in self-harming and suicide in adolescents. Lack of parent-adolescent communication, low levels of family cohesion and support, and family conflict were associated with adolescent suicidal ideation and DSH (33-35).

At the societal level, immigrant status has been considered a risk factor of adolescent suicide-related behaviors and DSH in different populations, mostly due to acculturation stress and insufficient support for immigrant youth. However, empirical findings are also inconclusive. Ponizovsky, Ritsner, and Modai (36) compared suicide ideation and suicide attempts among immigrant Jewish adolescents from the former Soviet Union to Israel and two indigenous samples of Jewish adolescents in Russia and in Israel. The results showed that the 6-month prevalence rate of suicidal ideation in the immigrant sample (10.9%) was significantly higher than that for Russian controls (3.5%) but not for Israeli natives (8.7%). On the other hand, an Australian study comparing native born Australians, Australian born children of immigrants, and immigrant adolescents did not find a higher risk of mental health problems among migrants (37). With reference to Chinese population, although there are reports showing that immigrant youth in Hong Kong did not display more problem behaviors, such as Internet addiction, than did local adolescents(38), no study has directly examined whether immigrant status is associated with adolescent suicide-related behaviors and deliberate self-harm.

While the identification of risk factors for a problem behavior is critical for prevention purpose, it is equally important to identify protective factors that diminish the risk of developing the problem. Positive youth development has been increasingly recognized as a significant protective factor for youth risk behaviors. Researchers have documented evidence that different positive youth development constructs are negatively related to a wide range of problem behaviors in adolescents, including drug abuse, delinquency, and Internet addiction (38-41). With reference to adolescent self-harm and suicidal behavior, several studies yielded associations of high self-esteem and high coping resources with low DSH. For example, McAuliffe et al (42) found that high self-esteem buffered the negative effect of passive-avoidant coping on self-harm. Kwok Lai and Shek (43) reported that suicidal ideation was positively related to hopelessness but negatively related to emotional competence and social problem solving in Hong Kong adolescents. These findings suggest that youth suicidal behaviors and DSH may be prevented by strengthening positive youth development. Based on a comprehensive literature review, 15 positive youth development constructs have been identified (44), including: bonding, resilience, social competence, recognition of positive behavior, emotional competence, cognitive competence, behavioral competence, moral competence, self-determination, self-efficacy, clear and positive identity, beliefs in the future, prosocial involvement, prosocial norms, and spirituality. However, there are no studies that directly examine the relationships between these constructs and adolescent DSH as well as suicide-related behavior.

Although a large amount of work has been done to examine the phenomenon of adolescent DSH and suicidal behaviors, there are several problems intrinsic to the current studies. First, existing findings on DSH and suicidal behavior among adolescents are inconclusive. This may be due to the inconsistent measurement tools and various definitions of DSH and suicidal behaviors used in different studies. For example, while self-harm behaviors without suicidal intention should be differentiated from those with suicidal intention, there are studies in which the two different types of self-harm were mixed together. Second, most existing studies are cross-sectional and retrospective in nature, which leaves the causality of the relationship between different psychosocial factors and DSH as well as suicidal behaviors undecided. Third, small or unrepresentative samples were frequently used. Reliable prevalence data from large and representative samples would help researchers to gain a more accurate picture of adolescent DSH and suicide. Fourth, in comparison to the abundant information on adolescent suicide and DSH in Western countries, evidence of the prevalence and correlates of the DSH and suicidal behaviors in Chinese adolescents is far from enough. Fifth, empirical studies investigating the role of positive youth development in adolescent DSH and suicide are almost non-existent.

Against the above background, the present study attempted to examine the prevalence and psychosocial correlates of deliberate self-harm and suicidal behaviors among Chinese adolescents based on a large and representative sample of secondary school students in Hong Kong. This chapter reports data collected at the first wave of a longitudinal study which aims at tracing youth development and determining the causal relationships between different psychosocial correlates and adolescent developmental outcomes. Deliberate self-harm was clearly differentiated from suicidal behaviors in terms of the existence of suicidal intention and a comprehensive measure which assesses various forms of self-harming behaviors was used. Suicidal behavior was operationally defined as the behaviors including suicide thoughts, suicide plan, and suicide attempt.

Specifically, our study focused on the following research questions: 1) what are the prevalence rates of DSH and suicidal behavior in Chinese adolescents in Hong Kong? 2) What are the relationships between gender, family economic status, family functioning, and Chinese adolescent DSH and suicide? Based the literature, the following hypotheses were proposed: a) females would have a higher level of DSH and suicidal behavior than did males; b) family economic status would be negatively related to adolescent DSH and suicidal behavior; c) family functioning would be negatively related to adolescent DSH and suicidal behavior. (3) What is the relationship between positive youth development constructs and DSH as well as suicidal behavior among Chinese adolescents? It is expected that there would be negative relationship between positive youth development and adolescent DSH and suicidal behavior.

OUR STUDY

Our study is part of a large longitudinal study aiming at tracing the development and risk behaviors among Hong Kong adolescents over time. A total of 28 secondary schools in Hong Kong were randomly selected to participate in the study, with 5 schools from Hong Kong Island, 7 schools from Kowloon, and 16 schools from New Territories. Data regarding self-harming and suicidal behaviors collected in the first wave of this study are analyzed in this paper.

All Secondary 1 students in the selected schools were invited to complete a questionnaire anonymously. There were 3,328 students responding to the questionnaire. The mean age of the participants was 12.59 years (SD = 0.74). These include 1,719 boys and 1,572 girls, with 37 students did not indicate their gender. While most students were born in Hong Kong (78.3%), there were 19.8% of the participants coming from Mainland China and 1.9% from other places. Among the participated students, most had parents who both had a job (56.6%), 32.9% had either father or mother being employed, and 10.5% had parents who were both unemployed. The background demographic information of the participants is summarized in Table 1.

In the school year of 2009-2010, the participants were invited to respond to a comprehensive youth development questionnaire including both existing instruments and scales developed by the first author. The questionnaire survey was conducted by a trained research assistant in classroom settings with standardized instructions.

At each measurement occasion, the purposes of the study were introduced and confidentiality of the data collected was repeatedly ensured to all participants. School, parental and student consent had been obtained before data collection. Participants responded to the questionnaires in a self-administered format. The research assistant was present throughout the administration process to answer possible questions from the participants.

Table 1. Descriptive statistics about participants

Categorical variables	n	%		
Gender				
Male	1,719	52.2%		
Female	1,572	47.8%		
Place of birth				
Hong Kong	2,590	78.3%		
Mainland China	655	19.8%		
Others	64	1.9%		
Parental marital status				
First marriage	2,781	84.4%		
Divorced	209	6.3%		
Separated	73	2.2%		
Remarried	129	3.9%		
Others (not first marriage)	104	3.2%		
Family economic status				
Receiving CSSA	225	6.8%		
Not receiving CSSA	2,606	78.3%		
Others	465	13.9%		
Continuous variables	Mean	SD	Range	Cronbach's α
Age	12.59	0.74	10-18	-
CFAIALL	3.73	0.81	1-5	0.90
CPYDS	4.51	0.70	1-6	0.96
ASC	3.12	0.67	1-5	0.67
CBC	4.45	0.75	1-6	0.87
PA	4.50	0.89	1-6	0.83
GPYDQ	4.50	0.71	1-6	0.93
PIT	4.24	0.96	1-6	0.87
DSH	0.04	0.10	0-1	0.83
SB	0.08	0.21	0-1	0.68

Notes: CSSA = Comprehensive Social Security Assistance; CFAIALL = general family interaction; CPYDS = positive youth development; ASC = academic school competence; CBC = cognitive behavioral competence; PA = prosocial attributes; GPYDQ = general positive youth development qualities; PIT = positive identity; DSH = deliberate self-harm; SB = suicidal behavior.

Participants were invited to respond to a composite questionnaire that comprises questions on demographic information, participants' family environment, family functioning, different measures of youth development constructs and problem behaviors. For family environment, participants responded to questions regarding parental presence, educational level, parental marital status and family economic status.

Family economic status is indexed by the question of whether the family of the participant is receiving Comprehensive Social Security Assistance (CSSA), a financial aid provided by Hong Kong Government for low-income populations, at the time of survey, with 1 = received CSSA and 0 = did not receive CSSA.

Students were also asked to indicate the marital status of their parents, including "divorced and not remarried", "separate and not remarried", "couple, first marriage", "couple, second or above marriage", and "others". The scales used to assess family functioning, deliberate self-harming behaviors, suicidal behaviors, and positive youth development constructs are introduced below. Internal consistency of each measure for the present sample is summarized in Table 1.

Assessment of family functioning

Nine items were designed to provide information about three aspects of the participants' family functioning, including family mutuality, family conflicts, and family communication. Students were asked to respond to a five-point Likert scale on their perceptions of different aspects in their family lives.

These items were abstracted from the Chinese Family Assessment Instrument (45). Average score across the nine items was used as the indicator of general family functioning, with high scores representing for high levels of family functioning. Reliability analysis showed that the scale was internally consistent (Cronbach's alpha = .90).

Deliberate self-harm behavior scale (DSHS)

This scale comprises 17 items that assess the occurrence of different deliberate self-harming behaviors of the participants in the past year, including cutting wrist, burning oneself, carving words or pictures into skin, scratching and biting oneself, rubbing sandpaper on body, dripping acid onto skin, using bleach or other chemical materials to scrub skin, sticking sharp objects and rubbing glass into skin, breaking bones, banging head against something to cause a bruise to appear, preventing wounds from healing, and other self-harm behaviors. Respondents answered yes (coded as 1) or no (coded as 0) to the 17 items according to their actual behavior in the past year.

To differentiate self-harming behaviors without suicidal intention from suicide-related behaviors, a note that the behavior shall be conducted without suicidal intention is emphasized in each item.

A composite score of DSHS was calculated for each individual by averaging the 17 item scores, which ranged from 0 to 1 with higher score representing more self-harm behaviors. Cronbach's alpha of the DSHS was 0.83 for the present sample.

Suicidal behavior scale (SBS)

Participants' suicidal behaviors were measured by a four-item SBS in terms of three aspects: suicidal thought, suicidal plan, and suicidal attempt. The first item measured suicidal thought, which asked about whether the respondents had seriously considered committing suicide in the past one year. The second item asked the participants whether they had made specific plan for suicide, i.e., suicidal plan. The third item enquired the number of actual suicide the participants had committed in the past year (0 = never; 1 = once to twice; 2 = three to four times; 3 = five to six times; 4 = seven to eight times; 5 = nine to ten times; 6 = more than ten times), i.e., suicidal attempts. For the present study, this item was recoded: 0 = never attempted suicide; 1 = attempted suicide at least once. If the participants reported having attempted suicide, they were asked to indicate whether their suicidal behaviors need medical treatment in the fourth item. A composite score of SBS was computed by averaging scores of item 1, item 2 and the recoded item 3, which represents for a general suicidal tendency of the participants. In this study, Cronbach's alpha for the three items was 0.68.

Chinese positive youth development scale (CPYDS)

The CPYDS consists of 15 subscales which are listed as follows:

1. Bonding Subscale (three items)
2. Resilience Subscale (three items)
3. Social Competence Subscale (three items)
4. Emotional Competence Subscale (three items)
5. Cognitive Competence Subscale (three items)
6. Behavioral Competence Subscale (three items)
7. Moral Competence Subscale (three items)
8. Self-Determination Subscale (three items)
9. Self-Efficacy Subscale (two items)
10. Beliefs in the Future Subscale (three items)
11. Clear and Positive Identity Subscale (three items)
12. Spirituality Subscale (three items)
13. Prosocial Involvement Subscale (three items)
14. Prosocial Norms Subscale (three items)
15. Recognition for Positive Behavior Subscale (three items)

Based on factor analyses, Shek and Ma (46) proposed that the 15 subscales in the CPYDS could be further reduced to four dimensions:

- Cognitive Behavioral Competence (CBC): Scale score was calculated by averaging scores on Cognitive Competence Subscale, Self-Determination Subscale, and Behavioral Competence Subscale.
- Prosocial Attributes (PA): Scale score was the mean score of Prosocial Involvement Subscale and Prosocial Norms Subscale.

- Positive Identity (PIT): Scale score was computed by averaging scores of Beliefs in the Future Subscale and Clear and Positive Identity Subscale.
- General Positive Youth Development Qualities (GPYDQ): Scale score was the mean score of Resilience Subscale, Social Competence Subscale, Self-Efficacy Subscale, Moral Competence Subscale, Bonding Subscale, Recognition for Positive Behavior Subscale, Spirituality Subscale, and Emotional Competence Subscale.

Both the overall score of CPYDS, calculated by averaging all item scores in the scale, and the above four composite indicators were used to assess participants' positive youth development in the present study. Scores of the five indicators all range from 1 to 6 with higher scores representing higher levels of competence in the constructs. Descriptive statistics about all variables under study are listed in Table 1. It should be noted that although the administered questionnaire includes other subscales of the CPYDS, findings regarding the subscales will be reported elsewhere. The present paper only focused on the predictive effects of the overall CPYDS score and the four second-order positive youth development constructs on adolescent self-harming and suicidal behavior. Cronbach's alpha coefficients were .96, .87, .83, .93, and .87 for the whole CPYDS, CBC subscale, PA subscale, GPYDQ subscale, and PIT subscale, respectively.

Academic and school competence scale

As a relatively independent positive youth development construct, participants' academic and school competence (ASC) were measured by three items. For the first item, participants were required to rate their perceived academic performance as compared to other peer students on a five-point Likert scale, with "1" = "very poor", "2" = "below average", "3" = "average", "4" = "above average", and "5" = "very good". The second item asked the extent to which the respondents were satisfied with their academic performance ("1" = "very dissatisfied", "2" = "dissatisfied", "3" = "neutral", "4" = "satisfied", and "5" = "very satisfied"). The last question asked the participants to rate their conduct in school on a five-point Likert scale ("1" = "very poor", "2" = "below average", "3" = "average", "4" = "above average", and "5" = "very good"). The ASC scale score was calculated by averaging the item scores and ranges from 1 to 5, with high scores representing for high academic and school competence. Reliability analysis showed that this measure was internally consistent (Cronbach's alpha = .67).

Data analytic plan

The first purpose of our study was to provide a descriptive profile of different self-harm and suicidal behaviors among Hong Kong adolescents. Therefore, numbers and percentages of adolescents who reported different self-harming behaviors and suicidal attempts were first computed. Means and standard deviations of two quantified indicators, DSH and SB, were also summarized and compared by groups of gender, immigrant status, parental marital status, and family economic status, which could offer a general picture of how self-harming and suicidal behaviors may vary across different groups.

Secondly, to investigate whether gender, age, immigration status, and positive youth development are predictive of adolescent self-harm and suicidal behaviors, two logistic regression models were tested using the probability of having self-harm behaviors and the probability of attempting suicide as the outcome variables, respectively. Specifically, basic demographic factors (age and gender) were entered in the first block; family economic status, parental marital status, and immigration status of the participant were entered into the second block; general family functioning was entered in the third block; and finally the participant's academic and school competence (ASC) and positive youth development (CPYDS) were entered into the fourth block. In the first model, whether the participants had displayed any of the listed self-harm behaviors served as the dependent variable. For the second model, the probability of showing any suicidal behavior (i.e., suicidal thinking, suicidal plan, or suicidal attempt) was the dependent variable. Because of the high correlations between CPYDS and different second-order positive youth development factors, two additional logistic regression analyses were conducted with the four second-order factors of positive youth development, including cognitive behavioral competence (CBC), prosocial attributes (PA), positive identity (PIT), and general positive youth development qualities (GPYDQ), being entered into the fourth block of the above regression models. The purpose was to examine the respective effects of different positive youth development constructs to adolescent self-harming and suicidal behaviors. It should be noted that while examining the relationship between immigration status and self-harm or suicidal behaviors, immigrant youth who were born in other places than mainland China was not included in the analyses because they only accounted for 1.9% of the participants. In other words, the present study focused on comparing local and immigrant adolescents from mainland China. In addition, as 465 participants did not indicate whether their family was receiving CSSA in the year of survey or not, they were not included in the regression analyses.

OUR FINDINGS

Numbers and percentages of participants who reported having different self-harm behaviors in the past one year are presented in Table 2, which provides a general picture of self-harm behaviors in Hong Kong adolescents. Several observations can be highlighted from the findings. First, self-harm behavior was common in Hong Kong adolescents.

Among the participated students, 1,087 respondents (32.7%) endorsed at least one form of deliberate self-harm behaviors in the past one year. Second, the most prevalent self-injurious behavior was "severely scratch oneself to the extent that scarring or bleeding occurred", reported by 10.4% of the participants. Other popular forms of self-injury included "intentionally prevent wounds from healing" (8.6%), "cut one's wrist, arms, or other areas of one's body" (8.3%), and "bite oneself to the extent that one's skin is broken" (7.4%). Third, severe self-harm behaviors, such as "break one's own bones" (0.6%), "drip acid onto one's skin" (0.3%), and "use bleach, comet, or oven cleaner to scrub one's skin" (0.5%), were relatively uncommon. Participants' suicidal behaviors in terms of suicide thought, suicide plan and suicide attempt are summarized in Table 3. Specifically, 13.7% of the adolescents

(N = 446) reported that they had seriously thought about attempting suicide; 4.9% (N = 158) had made specific suicidal plans, and 4.7% (N = 152) had actually attempted suicide during the past year. Of the 152 students who attempted suicide, approximately 15% reported that their attempts had resulted in an injury or poisoning that required medical treatment.

Table 2. Percentage of participants with self-harming behavior

During the past year, have you ever intentionally	No		Yes	
	Number	Percent	Number	Percent
1. Cut your wrist, arms, or other area(s) of your body?	3,042	91.7%	277	8.3%
2. Burned yourself with a cigarette?	3,297	99.2%	26	0.8%
3. Burned yourself with a lighter or a match?	3,274	98.7%	42	1.3%
4. Carved words into your skin?	3,153	95.1%	161	4.9%
5. Carved pictures, designs, or other marks into your skin?	3,135	94.9%	169	5.1%
6. Severely scratched yourself, to the extent that scarring or bleeding occurred?	2,956	89.6%	343	10.4%
7. Bit yourself, to the extent that you broke the skin?	3,045	92.6%	244	7.4%
8. Rubbed sandpaper on your body?	3,263	99.1%	30	0.9%
9. Dripped acid onto your skin?	3,279	99.7%	10	0.3%
10. Used bleach, comet, or oven cleaner to scrub your skin?	3,259	99.5%	16	0.5%
11. Stuck sharp objects such as needles, pins, staples, etc. into your skin (not including tattoos, ear piercing, needles used for drug use, or body piercing)?	3,158	96.8%	103	3.2%
12. Rubbed glass into your skin?	3,178	98.4%	52	1.6%
13. Broken your own bones?	3,203	99.4%	20	0.6%
14. Banged your head against something, to the extent that you caused a bruise to appear?	3,060	95.7%	138	4.3%
15. Punches yourself, to the extent that you caused a bruise to appear.	2,992	94.2%	184	5.8%
16. Prevented wounds from healing?	2,876	91.4%	272	8.6%
17. Done anything else to hurt yourself that was not asked about in this questionnaire?	2,986	95.3%	148	4.7%
Participants who had shown any of the above self-harm behaviors	**2,241**	**67.3%**	**1,087**	**32.7%**

Table 3. Percentage of participants with suicidal behavior in the past year

During the past one year	No		Yes	
	Number	Percent	Number	Percent
1. Have you seriously thought about attempting suicide?	2,816	86.3%	446	13.7%
2. Did you make a specific plan about how you would attempt suicide?	3,095	95.1%	158	4.9%
3. Did you actually make a suicide attempt?	3,095	95.3%	152	4.7%
4. If you attempted suicide, did that attempt result in an injury or poisoning that had to be treated by a doctor or nurse?	3,206	99.3%	22	0.7%
Participants who had shown any of the above suicidal behaviors	**2,758**	**85.3%**	**476**	**14.7%**

Psychosocial correlates of self-harm and suicidal behaviors

Means and standard deviations of DSH and SB in different groups of gender, immigrant status, parental marital status, and family economic status are first summarized in Table 4. T-tests and one way ANOVA were conducted to compare students' scores on DSH and SB among different groups. Several observations can be highlighted from the results. First, female students scored significantly higher than did male students in both DSH and SB, suggesting that girls were more likely to display self-harming and suicidal behaviors than were boys. Second, adolescents whose family receiving CSSA had relatively higher scores on SB than did students whose family did not receive CSSA, which indicates a possible role of low family economic status in adolescent suicidal behaviors. Third, local youth and immigrant adolescents did not differ in their DSH and SB scores. Fourth, parental marital status significantly predicted both DSH and SB. Post hoc analyses suggested that adolescents whose parents were divorced and remarried with other people scored significantly higher than did adolescents whose parent were married couple.

These results provide a rough picture of how different demographic factors may affect adolescent self-harming and suicidal behaviors.

Table 5 presents the simple correlations among family functioning, positive youth development constructs, DSH and SB. As predicted, general family functioning was negatively correlated with self-harming and suicidal behaviors, while positively correlated with all positive youth developmental indicators. Both the general indicator and different second-order factors of positive youth development were negatively correlated with self-harming behavior and suicide. These relationships were basically consistent with the literature and the hypotheses.

Table 4. Means and standard deviations of self-harm and suicidal behavior in different groups by gender, immigrant status, family economic status and parental marital status

	DSH				SB			
	Mean	SD	Statistics	*p*	Mean	SD	Statistics	*p*
Gender								
Male	.03	.10	$t = -2.23$	**.03**	.05	.14	$t = -5.40$	**.00**
Female	.04	.10			.08	.18		
Immigrant status								
Hong Kong	.04	.10	$t = -1.10$	.27	.07	.16	$t = 1.56$	.12
Mainland China	.03	.09			.06	.17		
Family economic status								
Not receiving CSSA	.04	.09	$t = 0.34$	.74	.06	.15	$t = 2.34$	**.02**
Receiving CSSA	.04	.10			.09	.19		
Parental marital status								
Divorced	.05	.13	$F = 4.48$	**.00**[a]	.07	.17	$F = 7.94$	**.00**[b]
Separated	.05	.09			.09	.19		
Married	.04	.09			.05	.15		
Remarried	.07	.13			.12	.22		
Others	.05	.12			.09	.19		

Note: [a] Tukey's HSD post hoc test showed that significant differences in DSH exist between married and remarried parental marital status.

[b] Tukey's HSD post hoc test showed that significant differences in SB exist between married and remarried parental marital status.

Table 5. Correlations among continuous variables

	CFAIALL	CPDYS	ASC	CBC	PA	GPYDQ	PIT	DSH
CFAIALL	-	-	-	-	-	-	-	-
CPDYS	.53	-	-	-	-	-	-	-
ASC	.28	.38	-	-	-	-	-	-
CBC	.37	.88	.26	-	-	-	-	-
PA	.42	.81	.28	.60	-	-	-	-
GPYDQ	.55	.97	.37	.79	.74	-	-	-
PIT	.42	.84	.40	.71	.63	.75	-	-
DSH	-.24	-.25	-.14	-.18	-.19	-.25	-.20	-
SB	-.26	-.24	-.13	-.14	-.19	-.26	-.18	.43

Note: CFAIALL = general family interaction; CPYDS = positive youth development; ASC = academic school competence; CBC = cognitive behavioral competence; PA = prosocial attributes; GPYDQ = general positive youth development qualities; PIT = positive identity; DSH = deliberate self-harm; SB = Suicidal behavior.

All correlations are significant at the 0.01 level.

The results of logistic regression analyses on self-harm behaviors (DSH) are shown in Table 6. There are several significant findings. First, gender predicted the probability of displaying self-destructive behaviors. The occurrence of self-injury was about 1.3 times higher among female students in comparison with male students (OR = 1.32, p = .01). Second, students who reported higher level of family functioning were less likely to show self-harm behaviors as compared to students whose family functioning was low (OR = 0.73, p < .001). Third, there was a negative relationship between participants' overall positive youth development and the occurrence of self-harm behaviors; the higher the positive youth development, the lower the risk of self-harm behaviors (OR = 0.72, p < .001). Fourth, higher academic and school competence was associated with lower occurrence of self-harm behaviors (OR = 0.79, p < .001).

To determine whether different aspects of positive youth development would contribute to adolescent self-harming behaviors differently, a separate regression model was tested with four second-order factors of positive youth development instead of CPYDS being entered into the fourth block of the initial model. As shown in Table 6, higher academic and school performance still predicted lower rates of self-harming behavior in this model (OR = 0.80, p = .01); general positive youth development qualities (GPYDQ) was negatively correlated with the occurrence of self-harm behaviors (OR = 0.55, p < .001). Unexpectedly, CBC positively contributed to DSH (OR = 1.26, p = .04), suggesting that there was an increase in the risk of self-injury in adolescents with higher cognitive behavioral competence.

Table 7 presents the results for the prediction of suicidal behavior (SB). First, adolescent girls were two times more likely to be engaged in suicidal behavior than did adolescent boys (OR = 2.07, p < .001). Second, the risk of suicide in adolescents whose parents were remarried with other persons was 2.53 times (p < .001) higher than adolescents from intact families.

Third, adolescents with higher academic and school competence (OR = 0.76, p = .01) demonstrated lower rate of risk for suicidal behavior. Fourth, higher overall positive youth development was associated with lower rate of suicidal behavior (OR = 0.55, p < .001).

Table 6. Logistic regression analyses on participants' self-harm behavior

	B	Odds Ratio	*p*
First block			
Age	0.07	1.07	.36
Gender	0.28	1.32	.01
Second block			
Immigration status	-0.13	0.88	.33
Family economic status (CSSA)	-0.18	0.83	.37
Parental marital status			
Parent_divorced	0.18	1.19	.41
Parent_separated	0.09	1.10	.79
Parent_remarried	0.18	1.20	.47
Parent_others	0.30	1.35	.29
Third block			
CFAALL	-0.31	0.73	.00
Fourth block			
ASC	-0.23	0.79	.00
CPYDS	-0.33	0.72	.00
Additional Analyses [a]	B	Odds Ratio	*p*
Fourth block			
ASC	-0.22	0.80	.01
CBC	0.23	1.26	.04
PA	-0.01	0.99	.90
GPYDQ	-0.60	0.55	.00
PIT	0.00	1.00	.97

Notes: [a] In additional analyses, four second-order factors of positive youth development (CBC, PA, GPYDQ and PIT) were used to replace CPYDS in the fourth block of the regression model. Other variables in the regression model and the order of entry were the same as the initial model.

Immigration status: 1 = immigrant from mainland China; 0 = local participant.

Family economic status: 1 = Receiving Comprehensive Social Security Assistance (CSSA); 2 = not receiving CSSA.

Parent_divorced: 1 = divorced; 0 = married (first marriage)

Parent_separated: 1 = separated; 0 = married (first marriage).

Parent_remarried: 1 = remarried; 0 = married (first marriage).

Parent_others: 1 = others (not first marriage); 0 = married (first marriage).

CFAIALL = general family interaction; ASC = academic school competence; CPYDS = positive youth development.

CBC = cognitive behavioral competence; PA = prosocial attributes; GPYDQ = general positive youth development; PIT = positive identity.

It should be noted that the effect of family economic status on suicidal behavior was non-significant in the regression model after other demographic variables being controlled. This suggests that the higher score of suicidal behavior in adolescents with lower family economic status found in the t-test results may be due to the moderating effects of other variables such as gender and parental marital status.

Results of the additional analyses also showed that higher levels of academic and school performance and general positive youth development qualities significantly predicted lower levels of suicidal behavior. In particular, the risk of suicidal behavior would decrease by approximately three times when participants' scores on general positive youth development increase one point (OR = 0.24, $p < .001$). This suggests that general positive youth development is a strong protective factor for adolescent suicide. Again, contrary to our expectation, higher cognitive and behavior competence was related to higher occurrence of suicidal behavior. The odds ratio was 1.94 ($p < .001$), which means that one point increased in the participant's cognitive behavioral competence score would almost double the risk of suicidal behavior for the participants.

Table 7. Logistic regression analyses on participants' suicidal behavior

	B	Odds Ratio	*p*
First block			
Age	-0.01	0.99	.95
Gender	0.73	2.07	.00
Second block			
Immigration status	-0.01	0.99	.95
Family economic status (CSSA)	0.34	1.41	.16
Parental marital status			
Parent_divorced	-0.09	0.92	.76
Parent_separated	-0.59	0.55	.24
Parent_remarried	0.93	2.53	.00
Parent_others	0.02	1.02	.95
Third block			
CFAIALL	-0.53	0.59	.00
Fourth block			
ASC	-0.27	0.76	.01
CPYDS	-0.60	0.55	.00
Additional Analyses [a]	B	Odds Ratio	*p*
Fourth block			
ASC	-0.26	0.77	.02
CBC	0.66	1.94	.00
PA	-0.05	0.95	.67
GPYDQ	-1.42	0.24	.00
PIT	0.09	1.09	.42

Notes: [a] In additional analyses, four second-order factors of positive youth development (CBC, PA, GPYDQ and PIT) were used to replace CPYDS in the fourth block of the regression model. Other variables in the regression model and the order of entry were the same as the initial model.

Immigration status: 1 = immigrant from mainland China; 0 = local participant.

Family economic status: 1 = Receiving Comprehensive Social Security Assistance (CSSA); 2 = not receiving CSSA.

Parent_divorced: 1 = divorced; 0 = married (first marriage)

Parent_separated: 1 = separated; 0 = married (first marriage)

Parent_remarried: 1 = remarried; 0 = married (first marriage).

Parent_others: 1 = others (not first marriage); 0 = married (first marriage).

CFAIALL = general family interaction; ASC = academic school competence; CPYDS = positive youth development.

CBC = cognitive behavioral competence; PA = prosocial attributes; GPYDQ = general positive youth development; PIT = positive identity.

Discussion

The present study explored the prevalence and psychosocial correlates of deliberate self-harm (DSH) and suicidal behavior among Chinese youth based on a large sample of Hong Kong secondary school students. The results suggested that both DSH and suicidal behavior were not rare among young people in Hong Kong. Several risk and protective factors were identified. First, being female and having remarried parents increased the likelihood of displaying DSH and suicidal behavior. Second, higher level of family functioning decreased the incidence of DSH and suicidal behavior. Third, academic and school competence and overall positive youth development were negatively related to the occurrences of both self-harming and suicidal behavior. These findings are basically consistent with our hypotheses and provide important information for developing evidence-based prevention strategies for DSH and suicidal behavior in Chinese adolescents.

In this study, 32.7% of the participants reported at least one form of DSH within the previous year. The prevalence rate was comparable to the figures reported in the United States (6,7) but it was apparently higher than in previous studies conducted among adolescents in different Chinese communities (47,48). This discrepancy might be an indicator for the increased incidence of DSH in Chinese youth. Another possible explanation may be that in contrast to previous studies, a more comprehensive measure of DSH that includes as many as 17 forms of self-harming behaviors was used in the present study, which perhaps increased the opportunity that various self-harming behaviors being disclosed. The prevalence of suicidal behaviors was found to be basically congruent with prior report. Around 13.7% of the adolescents reported having suicidal thoughts and 4.9% had suicidal plans in the past 12 months. It should be noted that among adolescents with suicidal plans (4.9%), almost all of them (4.7%) attempted suicide and 15% of the attempts were serious to the extent that medical treatment was required. These figures provide important information for helping professionals and policy makers in Hong Kong and other Chinese societies that DSH and suicidal behaviors are becoming an increasingly serious health problem for adolescents and thus timely intervention/prevention strategies are sorely needed.

Consistent with previous findings, adolescent girls were found to have significantly higher rates of DSH and suicidal behaviors than adolescent boys. Specifically, the occurrence of DSH was about 1.3 times higher among female students in comparison with male students; and girls were about 2.1 times more likely to show suicidal tendency. Most researchers have explained gender difference in DSH and suicidal behaviors in terms of the role of gender socialization experiences (49). For example, Clery argued that males learn to direct conflicts externally while women learn to turn their anger inward. As such, male aggression tends to be criminalized and female aggression tends to be expressed in the forms of internalized problems, such as self-injury (50). To further understand what factors may account for gender difference in DSH and suicide-related behavior in adolescents, the meaning of the two types of behaviors in the lives of male and female youth should be further investigated. It should be noted that although successful suicide has been found to occur more frequently in males than in females(51), the present study only focused on the less extreme forms of suicidal behaviors (unsuccessful suicide), i.e., suicidal thoughts, plans, and attempts. Further research is needed to examine gender difference in real suicide in Chinese adolescents.

Two family factors were found to have predictive effects on adolescent DSH and suicidal behavior: low level of family functioning (i.e., low family mutuality, low family communication and high family conflict) and having remarried parents increased the likelihood of these two kinds of risky behaviors. While there is abundant evidence supporting the protective role of good communication and harmonious relationships among family members for adolescent development (34), family conflict and parental marital discord have long turned out to be salient risk factors for emotional and behavioral problems in youth, because family conflict creates particularly stressful life experiences for children and adolescents (52,53). As a way of coping, adolescents use self-harm to release intense, overwhelming negative emotions and obtain a brief escape from the distress; to get a sense of control over the pain and their lives; and sometimes to deal with strong feelings of guilt, shame, or self-hatred (54). Desperate avoidance such as suicide and anger-based delinquency may also occur under such circumstances (55,56). In line with prior findings, the present results provide further support for the important role of family experiences in Chinese adolescents' self-harming and suicidal behaviors. Therefore, it seems necessary to involve units that target at improving various family factors in designing relevant prevention/intervention programs, such as building up supporting family relationships, reducing family conflicts, and providing support for different family members in non-intact family, especially children.

As expected, positive youth development significantly predicted DSH and suicidal behavior among Chinese adolescents. Higher levels of overall positive youth development and academic performance were closely related to lower rates of DSH and suicidal behaviors. The effects of positive youth development in adolescent promotion/prevention programs have been investigated by many researchers.

In the United States, Catalano et al. identified 25 effective programs focusing on positive youth development (44). These programs all demonstrated robust and sustained impacts on promoting positive outcomes and preventing problem behaviors (e.g., substance abuse, delinquency, campus violence, and youth pregnancy) among adolescents. In Hong Kong, Shek and colleagues (57) developed a multiple-year positive youth development program for Chinese adolescents, the Project P.A.T.H.S. After six years of implementation of the program in more than 200 secondary schools in Hong Kong, significant program effects were shown in multiple areas, including reduced adolescent problem behaviors (e.g., Internet addiction, delinquent behaviors, consumption of pornographic readings, and substance abuse) and increased positive developmental outcomes (e.g., bonding with others, emotional and social competence, self-efficacy, and prosocial norms) (39,41,58). Aligning with these findings, the present finding that positive youth development was negatively related to the likelihood of showing self-harming or suicidal behaviors provides direct support for the utilization of positive youth development programs in preventing adolescent risk behaviors.

Several unexpected findings were also observed. First, family economic status was related to neither adolescent DSH nor suicidal behavior. Second, immigrant students had no higher rates of DSH and suicidal behaviors than did local students.

These results seemed to be inconsistent with prior findings that that low family economic status and immigrant status often increased the vulnerability of self-harm and suicide in adolescents(59) due to the heightened exposure to multiple stressors (60), lack of material and social resources and support (61), and social exclusion caused by lack of family assets and/or immigrant identity (62).

One possible reason may be that family economic status was indexed by one item (i.e., whether the student was from a family with CSSA), so that the real economic condition of the family may not be fully reflected in the response. In future studies, multiple items and more quantitative measures of family economic status could be used. For immigrant status, it is possible that there are other variables moderating or mediating its effects on youth DSH and suicidal behaviors. Researchers have found that immigrant youth from China mainland to Hong Kong had higher levels of self-control, empathy, assertiveness and ability to read social cues which led to their better mental health than local youth (63).

To investigate which factors and how they affect the adaption of immigrant youth and prevent them from various risk behaviors could be a direction for future research.

Third, one positive youth development construct, cognitive and behavioral competence, was positively related to the occurrence of DSH and suicidal behavior. This finding is contradictory to the common finding that positive youth development helps to reduce problem behaviors. In this study, the measured cognitive and behavioral competence involves three aspects: cognitive competence, behavioral competence and a sense of self-determination. According to Catalano et al (44), while high levels of cognitive competence and behavioral competence enable one to develop skills for self-understanding, problem-solving, and making effective behavioral choices, a high sense of self-determination allows an individual to think for oneself and to take action consistent with that thought. In this sense, if people believe that self-harm or suicide could be an effective way to cope with painful events and to relieve one's sufferings, those with higher self-determination may be more likely to take real action, i.e. commit self-harming or suicidal behaviors.

This possibility can be further explored by separating self-determination from the general cognitive and behavioral competence and examining their respective relationships with different problem behaviors. On the other hand, the present finding also suggests that, to effectively prevent youth problem behaviors, different aspects/constructs of positive youth development must be developed concurrently. For example, when we try to foster a sense of self-determination in adolescents, we must also teach them skills that help to manage one's emotion (emotional competence), to adapt to change and stressful events in healthy and flexible ways (resilience), and to develop commitment to social relationships in the family, school, and culture (bonding). The interactive effects among different positive youth development constructs on preventing adolescent risk behaviors could be tested in future research.

This study examined the prevalence of deliberate self-harm (DSH) and suicidal behaviors among Chinese adolescents based on empirical research. The high prevalence of DSH and suicidal behavior in Hong Kong secondary school students could be considered a forewarning to researchers, school practitioners, and public health professionals in Hong Kong society, and perhaps in other Chinese communities. Several correlates of the two phenomena were identified, including gender, family functioning, parental marital status, academic and school competence, and positive youth development.

Such knowledge is useful to help researchers and professionals better understand, predict, prevent and treat DSH and suicidal behaviors among Chinese adolescents. In addition, the fact that DSH and suicidal behavior shared similar associated factors provides further support for the preventive approach that addresses both risk and protective factors for multiple problems simultaneously, such as the Project P.A.T.H.S.

Acknowledgments

The preparation for the study and this chapter and the Project P.A.T.H.S. were financially supported by The Hong Kong Jockey Club Charities Trust.

References

[1] Nock MK, Joiner Jr TE, Gordon KH, Lloyd-Richardson E, Prinstein MJ. Non-suicidal self-injury among adolescents: diagnostic correlates and relation to suicide attempts. Psychiatr Res 2006;30: 65-72.

[2] Posner K, Oquendo MA, Gould M, Stanley B, Davies M. Columbia Classification Algorithm of Suicide Assessment (C-CASA): classification of suicidal events in the FDA's pediatric suicidal risk analysis of antidepressants. Am J Psychiatr 2007;164:1035-43.

[3] Silverman MM, Berman AL, Sanddal ND, O'Carroll PW, Joiner TE. Rebuilding the tower of Babel: a revised NSSI and suicide attempts nomenclature for the study of suicide and suicidal behaviors. Part 2: suicide-related ideations, communications and behaviors. Suicide Life Threat Behav 2007;37:264-77.

[4] Hawton K, Rodham K, Evans E, Weatherall R. Deliberate self harm in adolescents: self report survey in schools in England. BMJ 2002;325: 1207-11.

[5] Ross S, Heath N. A study of the frequency of self mutilation in a community sample of adolescents. J Youth Adolesc 2002;31:67-77.

[6] Gratz KL. Measurement of deliberate self-harm: preliminary data on the Deliberate Self-Harm Inventory. J. Psychopathol Behav Assess 2001;23: 253-63.

[7] Jacobson CM, Gould M. The epidemiology and phenomenology of non-suicidal self-injurious behavior among adolescents: a critical review of the literature. Arch Suicide Res 2007;11:129-47.

[8] Whitlock J, Eckenrode J, Silverman D. Self-injurious behaviors in a college population. Pediatrics 2006;117:1939-48.

[9] Gollust S, Eisenberg D, Golberstein E. Prevalence and correlates of self-injury among university students. J Am Coll Health 2008;56: 491-8.

[10] Favaro A, Ferrara S, Santonastaso P. Self-injurious behavior in a community sample of young women: relationship with childhood abuse and other types of self- damaging behaviors. J Clin Psychiatr 2007;68:122-31.

[11] Zoroglu SS, Tuzun U, Sar V, Tutkun H, Savaçs HA, Ozturk M, et al. Suicide attempts and self-mutilation among Turkish high school students in relation with abuse, neglect, and dissociation. Psychiatry Clin Neurosci 2003;57:119-26.

[12] Fliege H, Lee J, Grimm A, Lapp BF. Risk factors and correlates of deliberate self-harm behavior: a systematic review. J Psychosomatic Res 2009;66:477-93.

[13] Kessler RC, Borges G, Walters EE. Prevalence of and risk factors for lifetime suicide attempts in the National Comorbidity Survey. Arch Gen Psychiatry 1999;56:617-26.

[14] Rey GC, Narring F, Ferron C, Michaud PA. Suicide attempts among adolescents in Switzerland: prevalence, associated factors and comorbidity. Acta Psychiatr Scand 1998;98:28-33.

[15] Evans E, Hawton K, Rodham K, Deeks J. The prevalence of suicidal phenomena in adolescents: a systematic review of population-based studies. Suicide Life Threat Behav 2005;35:239-49.

[16] Liu X, Sun Z, Yang Y. Parent-reported suicidal behavior and correlates among adolescents in China. J Affect Disord 2008;105:73-80.

[17] Tang J, Yu Y, Wu Y, Du Y, Ma Y, Zhu H, Zhang P, Liu Z. Association between non-suicidal self-injuries and suicide attempts in Chinese adolescents and college students: a cross-section study. PLoS. One 2011;6:e17977 (epub ahead of print). doi:10.1371/journal.pone.0017977.

[18] Liu XC. Sleep and adolescent suicidal behavior. Sleep 2004;27:1351-8.

[19] Pan X, Zhang C, Shi Z. Soft drink and sweet food consumption and suicidal behaviours among Chinese adolescents. Acta Paediatr 2011 (epub ahead of print). doi: 10.1111/j.1651-2227.2011.02369.x.

[20] Chan W, Law C, Liu K, Wong P, Law Y, Yip P. Suicidality in Chinese adolescents in Hong Kong: the role of family and cultural influences. Soc Psychiatry Psychiatr Epidemiol 2009;44:278-84.

[21] Brunner R, Parzer P, Haffner J, Steen R, Roos J, Klett M, Resch F. Prevalence and psychological correlates of occasional and repetitive deliberate self-harm in adolescents. Arch Pediatr Adolesc Med 2007;161:641-9.

[22] Kirkcaldy BD, Brown J, Siefen R. Disruptive behavioural disorders, self harm and suicidal ideation among German adolescents in psychiatric care. Int J Adolesc Med Health 2006;18:597-614.

[23] Lipschitz D, Winegar R, Nicolaou A, Hartnick E, Wolfson M, Southwick S. Perceived abuse and neglect as risk factors for suicidal behavior in adolescent inpatients. J Nerv Ment Dis 1999;187:32-9.

[24] Kapur N, Cooper J, King-Hele S, Webb R, Lawlor M, Rodway C, Appleby L. The repetition of suicidal behavior: a multicenter cohort study. J Clin Psychiatry 2006;67:1599-1609.

[25] Schmidtke A, Bille-Brahe U, DeLeo D, Kerkhof A, Bjerke T, Crepet P, et al. Attempted suicide in Europe: rates, trends and sociodemographic characteristics of suicide attempters during the period 1989-1992. Results of the WHO/EURO multicentre study on parasuicide. Acta Psychiatr Scand 1996;93:327-38.

[26] Blumental SJ, Kupfer DJ. Suicide over the life cycle. Washington, DC: American Psychiatric Press, 1990.

[27] Stillion JM, McDowell EE, May JH. Suicide across the life span—premature exits. New York: Hemisphere, 1989.

[28] Chan W, Law CK, Liu KY, Wong P, Law YW, Yip P. Suicidality in Chinese adolescents in Hong Kong: the role of family and cultural influences. Soc Psychiatry Psychiatr Epidemiol 2009;44:278-84.

[29] Hesketh T, Ding QJ, Jenkins R. Suicide ideation in Chinese adolescents. Soc Psychiatry Psychiatr Epidemiol 2002;37:230-5.

[30] Wong JPS, Stewart SM, Ho SY, Lam TH. Risk factors associated with suicide attempts and other self-injury among Hong Kong adolescents. Suicide Life Threat Behav 2007;37:453-66.

[31] Sourander A, Aromaa M, Pihlakoski L, Haavisto A, Rautava P, Helenius H, et al. Early predictors of deliberate self-harm among adolescents. A prospective follow-up study from age 3 to age 15. J Affect Disord 2006;93:87-96.

[32] Derouin A, Bravender T. Living on the edge: the current phenomenon of self-mutilation in adolescents. Am J Matern Child Nurs 2004;29:12-8.

[33] Portzky G, de Wilde EJ, van Heeringen K. Deliberate self-harm in young people: differences in prevalence and risk factors between the Netherlands and Belgium. Eur Child Adolesc Psychiatry 2008;17:179-86.

[34] Stivers C. Parent-adolescent communication and its relationship to adolescent depression and suicide proneness. Adolescence 1998;23:291-5.

[35] Syed EU, Khan MM. Pattern of deliberate self-harm in young people in Karachi, Pakistan. Crisis 2008;29:159-63.

[36] Ponizovsky AM, Ritsner MS, Modai I. Suicidal ideation and suicide attempts among immigrant adolescents from the former Soviet Union to Israel. J Am Acad Child Adolesc Psychiatry 1999;38:1433-41.

[37] Klimidis S, Stuart G, Minas IH, Ata AW. Immigrant status and gender effects on psychopathology and self-concept in adolescents: a test of the migration-morbidity hypothesis. Compr. Psychiatry 1994;35:393-404.

[38] Shek DTL, Yu L. Internet addiction in Hong Kong adolescents: profiles and psychosocial correlates. Int J Disabil Hum Dev 2012;11:133-42.

[39] Sun RCF, Shek DTL. Positive youth development, life satisfaction and problem behavior among Chinese adolescents in Hong Kong: a replication. Soc Indic Res 2012;105:541-59.

[40] Shek DTL. Positive youth development and behavioral intention to gamble among Chinese adolescents in Hong Kong. Int J Adolesc Med Health 2010;22:163-72.

[41] Shek DTL, Yu L. Prevention of adolescent problem behavior: longitudinal impact of the Project P.A.T.H.S. in Hong Kong. ScientificWorldJournal 2011;11:546-67.
[42] McAuliffe C, Corcoran P, Keeley HS, Arensman E, Bille-Brahe U, De Leo D, et al. Problem-solving ability and repetition of deliberate self-harm: a multicentre study. Psychol Med 2005;35:1-11.
[43] Kwok SYC, Shek DTL. Social problem solving, family functioning and suicidal ideation among Chinese adolescents in Hong Kong. Adolescence 2009;44:391-406.
[44] Catalano RF, Berglund ML, Ryan JAM, Lonczak HS, Hawkins JD. Positive youth development in the United States: research findings on evaluations of positive youth development programs. Prev Treat 2002;5:1-111.
[45] Shek DTL, Ma CMS. The Chinese Family Assessment Instrument (C-FAI): hierarchical confirmatory factor analyses and factorial invariance. Soc Indic Res 2010;20:112-23.
[46] Shek DTL, Ma CMS. Dimensionality of the Chinese Positive Youth Development Scale: confirmatory factor analyses. Soc Indic Res 2010;98:41-59.
[47] Li YM. Deliberate self-harm and relationship to alcohol use at an emergency department in eastern Taiwan. Kaohsiung J Med Sci 2007;23:247-53.
[48] You J, Leung F, Fu K, Lai CM. The prevalence of nonsuicidal self-injury and different subgroups of self-injurers in Chinese adolescents. Arch Suicide Res 2011;15:75-86.
[49] Frost M. Self-harm and the social work relationship. Soc Work Monogr 1995;134.
[50] Clery C. Self-directed violence in adolescence: a psychotherapeutic perspective. In: Boswell G, ed. Violent children and adolescents: asking the question why. London: Whurr, 2000:91-103.
[51] Branje SJT, van Doorn M, van der Valk I, Meeus W. Parent-adolescent conflicts, conflict resolution types, and adolescent adjustment. J Appl Dev Psychol 2009;30:195-204.
[52] Schraedley PK, Gotlib IH, Hayward C. Gender differences in correlates of depressive symptoms in adolescents. J Adolesc Health 1999;25:98-108.
[53] Turner HA, Finkelhor D, Ormrod R. The effect of lifetime victimization on the mental health of children and adolescents. Soc Sci Med 20006;62:13-27.
[54] Agnew R. Pressured into crime: an overview of general strain theory. Los Angeles, CA: Roxbury, 2006.
[55] Crowell SE, Beauchaine TP, McMauley E, Smith CJ, Vasilev CA, Stevens AL. Parent-child interactions, peripheral serotonin, and self-inflicted injury in adolescents. J Consult Clin Psychol 2008;76:15-21.
[56] Gladstone GL, Parker GB, Mitchell PB, Malhi GS, Wilhelm K, Austin MP. Implications of childhood trauma for depressed women: an analysis of pathways from childhood sexual abuse to deliberate self-harm and revictimization. Am J Psychiatr 2004;161:1417-25.
[57] Shek DTL, Ma HK, eds. Special issue: evaluation of the Project P.A.T.H.S.: replications. ScientificWorldJournal 2010;10:178-272.
[58] Shek DTL, Ma CMS. Impact of the Project P.A.T.H.S. in the junior secondary school years: individual growth curve analyses. ScientificWorldJournal 2011;11:253-66.
[59] Beautrais AL, Joyce PR, Mulder RT. Risk factors for serious suicide attempts among youths aged 13 through 24 years. J Am Acad Child Adolesc Psychiat 1996;35:1174-82.
[60] McLeod JD, Shanahan MJ. Trajectories of poverty and children's mental health. J Health Soc Behav 1996;37:207-20.
[61] Eamon MK, Zuehl RM. Maternal depression and physical punishment as mediators of the effect of poverty on socioemotional problems of children in single-mother families. Am J Orthopsychiat 2001;71:218-26.
[62] von Reuden U, Gosch A, Rajmil L, Bisegger C, Ravens-Sieberer U. Socioeconomic determinants of health related quality of life in childhood and adolescence: results from a European study. J Epidemiol Commun Health 2006;60:130-5.
[63] Wong FKD, Yan P, Lo E, Hung M. Mental health and social competence of mainland Chinese immigrant and local youth in Hong Kong: a comparison. J Ethnic Cult Divers Soc Work 2003;12:85-110.

In: Adolescence and Behavior Issues in a Chinese Context ISBN: 978-1-62618-614-9
Editors: DTL Shek, RCF Sun and Joav Merrick

Chapter 9

ASSESSMENT OF PROBLEM GAMBLING IN A CHINESE CONTEXT

Daniel TL Shek, PhD, FHKPS, BBS, JP*[*][1-5] and Elda ML Chan[6]

[1]Department of Applied Social Sciences,
The Hong Kong Polytechnic University, Hong Kong, PRC
[2] Centre for Innovative Programmes for Adolescents and Families,
Department of Applied Social Sciences,
The Hong Kong Polytechnic University, Hong Kong, PRC
[3]Department of Social Work, East China Normal University,
Shanghai, PRC
[4]Kiang Wu Nursing College of Macau, Macau, PRC
[5]Division of Adolescent Medicine, Department of Pediatrics,
Kentucky Children's Hospital, University of Kentucky College
of Medicine, Lexington, KY, US
[6]Even Centre, Tung Wah Group of Hospitals, Hong Kong, PRC

ABSTRACT

There is a severe lack of instruments assessing problem gambling in Chinese people. This chapter examined the psychometric properties of the Chinese version of the Maroondah Assessment Profile for Problem Gambling (Chinese G-MAP) based on the responses of eight problem gamblers and 125 pathological gamblers seeking help from a problem gambling treatment centre. Reliability analyses showed that the G-MAP and its related domains and scales were generally internally consistent. There are also several lines of evidence suggesting that the Chinese G-MAP and the various domains are valid: a) the various G-MAP domain and scale measures were significantly correlated among themselves; b) the G-MAP measures were significantly correlated with pathological gambling behavior assessed by the DSM-IV; c) the G-MAP total scale and domain measures were able to discriminate problem gamblers and pathological gamblers. The

[*] Correspondence: Professor Daniel T.L. Shek, PhD, FHKPS, BBS, JP, Chair Professor of Applied Social Sciences, Faculty of Health and Social Sciences, Department of Applied Social Sciences, The Hong Kong Polytechnic University, Room HJ407, Core H, Hunghom, Hong Kong. E-mail: daniel.shek@polyu.edu.hk.

present study suggests that the Chinese G-MAP possesses acceptable psychometric properties that can be used in research and practice settings.

INTRODUCTION

A survey of the literature shows that pathological gambling is a growing problem in the global context. Based on the existing prevalence studies of problem gambling in the United States, Petry (1) reported the prevalence rates of pathological gambling was around 1% to 2% of the general population, whereas sub-threshold pathological gambling was around 3% to 4% of the general population. In Canada, Cox, Yu, Afifi and Ladouceur (2) conducted a survey of the prevalence rates across 10 Canadian provinces and reported that the 12-month prevalence of gambling problems in Canada was 2.0% with variations across different provinces. In Spain, Becona (3) reported lifetime and past year prevalence rates of pathological gambling were 0.92% and 0.31%, respectively. Findings on the prevalence rates of pathological gambling in Sweden and New Zealand have also been reported (4).

There are also research studies suggesting that problem gambling is a growing problem in Hong Kong. The Centre for Social Policy Studies of the Department of Applied Social Sciences and the General Education Centre of The Hong Kong Polytechnic University (5) conducted a ground-breaking study of gambling among the general public in Hong Kong. Using the DSM-IV criteria for assessing pathological gambling, the researchers found that 1.85% of the 2,004 respondents could be classified as "probable pathological gamblers" (i.e., respondents displaying 5 or more symptoms). Fong and Ozorio (6) conducted the first scientific study on pathological gambling in Macau. Utilizing computer-assisted random digit dialing method (N = 1,121 interviews), results showed that 1.78% and 2.5% of the respondents could be classified as probable pathological gamblers and problem pathological gamblers, respectively.

What are the factors leading to problem gambling? With reference to the ecological models, an integration of the theories and research findings in the literature shows that several groups of factors would increase the likelihood of pathological gambling.

In the first place, there are theories suggesting that cognitive biases and distortions contribute to the development of pathological gambling. For example, many pathological gamblers believe that they can beat the gambling industry and they will win despite repeated loss.

Empirically, many studies have showed that experience of illusion of control and unrealistic perception of luck are prevalent in problem gamblers (7). Secondly, emotional factors are related to problem gambling. There are theories suggesting that gambling was consciously or unconsciously used as a strategy to cope with negative emotions in pathological gamblers. There are also research findings showing that there were greater emotional problems (depression, suicidal ideation) in adolescent gamblers (8), and there was high impulsivity in adolescent problem gamblers (9). Dickson, Derevensky and Gupta (10) also reported heightened risk for suicidal ideation and attempts in problem gamblers.

Third, situational factors are related to problem gambling. There are theories suggesting that inability to cope with demands in life contributes to pathological gambling. Research studies have showed that the coping behavior in adolescent gamblers was poor (8) and that problem gambling may occur after negative life events. There are also studies showing that resilience was negatively related to adolescent high risk behavior.

Fourth, there are theories suggesting that negative self-perceptions and low self-image (i.e., attitudinal factors) were intrinsic to pathological gambling. As such, pathological gamblers may make use of gambling to obtain achievement. There are research findings showing that adolescent gambling was closely related to delinquency and conduct problems which would strengthen the negative image of pathological gamblers (11). Lower self-esteem in adolescent problem gamblers was also reported (10).

Finally, there are theories suggesting that interpersonal and social problems are conducive to pathological gambling. For example, many parents and friends of adolescent gamblers were gamblers. There are also research findings showing that perceived family and peer support were poor among adolescent problem gamblers (11) and quality friendships and relationships were lost and replaced by gambling associates in pathological gamblers (12). Finally, it was found that there was higher susceptibility to peer pressure in probable pathological gamblers (9).

Obviously, a careful assessment of the above factors in problem gamblers would be important to give a clear picture about the possible factors that are conducive to the problem and the related assessment would give pointers to intervention and prevention at different levels.

In this study, the psychometric properties of the Chinese version of the Maroondah Assessment Profile for Problem Gambling (Chinese G-MAP) based on the work of Loughnan, Pierce and Sagris-Desmond (13) would be examined.

There are 5 domains and 17 scales in the G-MAP that resemble the five groups of factors related to pathological gambling outlined above. The domains and related scales of the G-MAP are as follows:

Domain 1: Beliefs about Winning Domain (Cognitive Problems)

- Control Scale: belief in the efficacy of one's system
- Prophecy Scale: use of intuition and ideas about luck to achieve successful outcomes
- Uninformed Scale: belief that gambling is a reasonable way to make money

Domain 2: Feelings Domain (Emotional Problems)

- Good Feelings Scale: use of gambling to lift one's mood
- Boredom Scale: use of gambling to alleviate boredom
- Numbness Scale: dissociation and disconnection from emotional responses when engaging in gambling
- Relaxation Scale: use of gambling to control stress

Domain 3: Situations Domain (Life Situations Related to Pathological Gambling)

- Desperation: gambling as a result of financial desperation
- Transition: relationship between gambling and transitional events in lives

- Oasis: gambling behavior as an "escape" from the perceived demands in life (coping problem)
- Mischief: gambling as a result of the dire to be "naughty" or rebellious

Domain 4: Attitudes to Self Domain (Self-Concept and Psychological Problem)

- Negative Life-Script: belief that others see one as a "loser" and wish that gambling can help them to be a "winner"
- Entrenchment: belief that gambling is a disease or affliction that can only be solved by life long abstinence
- Self Harm: conscious use of gambling to punish or hurt oneself
- Winner Life-Script: gambling as a result of the desire to maintain self-image of being a "winner"

Domain 5: Social Domain (Social Influences)

- Friendship: use of gambling to increase social encounter
- Shyness: use of gambling to satisfy the desire to be around people but minimize the pressure to interact with them

Based on the responses of Chinese problem and pathological gamblers to the Chinese G-MAP, the psychometric properties of the Chinese G-MAP were examined in this study.

There are two questions addressed in this study: 1) Are the Chinese G-MAP measures internally consistent? 2) Is the Chinese G-MAP valid? For the second question, the following information would be examined: a) inter-relationships among the G-MAP measures and scales; b) correlation between the G-MAP measures and pathological gambling behavior assessed by the DSM-IV; c) the ability of the G-MAP total scale and domain measures to discriminate problem gamblers and pathological gamblers.

OUR WORK

Our study was based on the clients seeking help from the Even Centre, Tung Wah Group of Hospitals (N = 134).

When these clients sought help from the Even Centre, they were requested to complete a questionnaire with the following sections:

1. Demographic information (e.g., gender, age, and marital status)
2. Presenting problems (e.g., gambling problem, occupational problem, suicidal behavior and interpersonal problems)
3. Problems arising from the debts
4. Whether family members and friends are helping the client's to pay off his debts
5. Employment status
6. Source of income
7. Monthly income

8. Age of first gambling
9. Gambling age (i.e., duration of gambling)
10. Duration of problem gambling
11. Gambling activities leading to gambling problems
12. Current gambling situation
13. Gambling history
14. Family background and structure
15. Personal background and developmental history
16. Health and mental health conditions
17. Whether receiving psychiatric treatment
18. Risk assessment
19. Problem behavior (e.g., substance abuse, the Net addiction, criminal history)
20. Self-assessment of gambling problem
21. Assessment based on the G-MAP
22. Proposed treatment plan

Besides the above self-report questionnaire, the participants were also assessed by the workers using the diagnostic criteria for pathological gambling based on the 4th Edition of the Diagnostic and Statistical Manual of Mental Disorders (DSM-IV). If a participant endorsed 3 to 4 criteria, he/she was considered to have problem gambling. If a participant endorsed five or more criteria, the person was regarded to have pathological gambling.

The client was also requested to complete the Chinese G-MAP. The G-MAP is an 85-item self-report inventory that assesses 17 aspects associated with problem gambling. The derivation of the 17 aspects of the tool was based on the clinical experiences and related discussion of the three clinicians who developed the tool (13). According to the test developers, the related 17 scales could be further grouped into five domains.

The psychometric properties of the Chinese G-MAP were examined in this study. For the reliability of the tool, the internal consistency of the G-MAP total scale, five domain scales and the 17 individual scales were examined. For the validity of the G-MAP measures, it was expected that different G-MAP domains and scales would have significant correlations among themselves. As the G-MAP measures (e.g., biased beliefs about gambling) are theoretically related to gambling behavior assessed by the diagnostic criteria of the DSM-IV, it would be expected that the G-MAP measures would be significantly related to the DSM-IV assessment scores (i.e., construct validity). Finally, based on the classification of gamblers using the DSM-IV, it would be expected that different types of gamblers would have different scores on the G-MAP measures (i.e. criterion-related validity).

WHAT WE FOUND

Based on the operational definition that those who endorsed five or more symptoms were regarded as "pathological gamblers", 94.0% of the respondents (N = 125) could be regarded as pathological gamblers and 6% of them (N = 8) could be regarded as problem gamblers.

Concerning the reliability of the Chinese G-MAP, the findings showed that the G-MAP measures were basically internally consistent (Table 1). With reference to the 85-item

Chinese G-MAP, results showed that the scale was internally consistent (alpha = .96 and mean inter-item correlation = .21). With the exception of items 4, 7, 38 and 55, the values of the item-total correlation coefficients were acceptable. For the different G-MAP domains, the domain scales were internally consistent.

For the validity of the G-MAP, there are several lines of evidence suggesting that the tool and the related measures are reliable. First, assuming that the scales in each domain are assessing similar traits, it would be expected that the different scales and domains would be inter-related. The findings are basically consistent with this general expectation. The relevant findings are presented in Table 2. Second, based on the predictions of different models, it would be expected that there would be inter-relationships amongst the G-MAP domains. The related findings are presented in Table 3.

Table 1. Coefficient Alpha and Mean Item-item Correlation Coefficient for the G-MAP Domains and Scales

Measures	Coefficient Alpha
• Beliefs about Winning Domain	.62
• Control Scale	.87
• Prophecy Scale	.69
• Uninformed Scale	.82
• Feelings Domain	.82
• Good Feelings Scale	.80
• Relaxation Scale	.75
• Boredom Scale	.83
• Numbness Scale	.57
• Situations Domain	.82
• Oasis Scale	.73
• Transition Scale	.83
• Desperation Scale	.73
• Mischief Scale	.73
• Attitudes to Self Domain	.68
• Negative Life-script Scale	.78
• Winner Life-script Scale	.70
• Entrenchment Scale	.42
• Harm to Self Scale	.66
• Social Domain	.83
• Friendship Scale	.68
• Shyness Scale	.72
G-MAP	.96

Third, using pathological gambling defined by the DSM-IV (14) as the criterion measure, findings showed that the G-MAP scores were generally correlated with the DSM-IV scores (see Table 4 and Table 5). Finally, the findings in Table 6 showed that with the exception of some individual scales, the scale, domain and total scale measures of the Chinese G-MAP were able to discriminate pathological gamblers and problem gamblers.

Table 2. Inter-relationships of the G-MAP scales in each domain

Domain 1	Control		Prophecy		Uniformed		
Control	1						
Prophecy	.29	**	1				
Uniformed	.39	***	.42	***	1		
Domain 2	**Good feelings**		**Boredom**		**Numbness**		**Relaxation**
Good feelings	1						
Boredom	.59	***	1				
Numbness	.43	***	.33	***	1		
Relaxation	.77	***	.57	***	.47	***	1
Domain 3	**Desperation**		**Transition**		**Oasis**		**Mischief**
Desperation	1						
Transition	.51	***	1				
Oasis	.49	***	.61	***	1		
Mischief	.40	***	.54	***	.71	***	1
Domain 4	**Negative Life-Script**		**Entrenchment**		**Self Harm**		**Winner Life-Script**
Negative Life-Script	1						
Entrenchment	.21	*	1				
Self Harm	.35	***	.07	ns	1		
Winner Life-Script	.70	***	.26	**	.35	***	1
Domain 5	**Friendship**		**Shyness**				
Friendship	1						
Shyness	.72	***	1				

* p < .05; ** p < .01; *** p < .001; ns non-significant.

DISCUSSION

As far as the reliability of the G-MAP measures is concerned, the internal consistency of the G-MAP total scale, 5 domain scales and the 17 individual scales was generally established in the present study. With the exception of the Numbness Scale and Entrenchment Scale, the inter-item correlation, item-total correlation and coefficient alpha statistics related to each measure were acceptable (15). In line with our expectation, the G-MAP domains and scales were significantly correlated among themselves. This observation suggests that the cognitive, emotional, attitudinal and interpersonal factors are inter-related. In the long run, it would be theoretically interesting to examine the inter-relationships among the different domains.

Table 3. Correlations amongst the G-MAP domain measures

	Beliefs about Winning Domain		Feelings Domain		Situations Domain		Attitudes to Self Domain		Social Domain		G-MAP
Beliefs about Winning Domain	1										
Feelings Domain	.39	***	1								
Situations Domain	.54	***	.67	***	1						
Attitudes to Self Domain	.65	***	.66	***	.77	***	1				
Social Domain	.48	***	.68	***	.68	***	.69	***	1		
G-MAP	.71	***	.84	***	.90	***	.90	***	.82	***	1

* $p < .05$; ** $p < .01$; *** $p < .001$; ns non-significant.

Table 4. Correlation coefficients on the relationships between the Chinese G-MAP measures and the DSM-IV measures

Measure	DSM-IV Total Score		DSM-IV Classification Score	
Control	.10	ns	.14	ns
Prophecy	.08	ns	.12	ns
Uninformed	.31	***	.33	***
Good feelings	.26	**	.16	ns
Boredom	.24	**	.17	*
Numbness	.10	ns	-.04	ns
Relaxation	.26	**	.21	*
Desperation	.46	***	.26	**
Transition	.26	**	.18	*
Oasis	.31	***	.18	*
Mischief	.27	**	.08	ns
Negative Life-Script	.17	*	.17	*
Entrenchment	.20	*	.11	ns
Self Harm	.06	ns	-.10	ns
Winner Life-Script	.17	*	.19	*
Friendship	.27	**	.23	**
Shyness	.28	**	.19	*
G-MAP	.34	***	.24	***

* p < .05; ** p < .01; *** p < .001; ns non-significant.

Table 5. Correlation coefficients on the relationships between the Chinese G-MAP domain measures and the DSM-IV measures

Measure	DSM-IV Total Score		DSM-IV Classification Score	
Beliefs about Winning Domain	.21	*	.26	**
Feelings Domain	.27	**	.16	ns
Situations Domain	.40	***	.22	*
Attitudes to Self Domain	.21	*	.15	ns
Social Domain	.29	**	.23	**

* p < .05; ** p < .01; *** p < .001; ns non-significant.

For the micro-theories, it would be expected that inner problems (e.g., cognitive problems) would be precursors of situational problems (e.g., desperation). On the other hand, extra-individual theories would predict that environmental problems (e.g., family issues) would lead to inner problems. Consistent with the expectation that the G-MAP measures would be significantly related to the DSM-IV scores, the findings showed that there was a general relationship between these two domains, thus providing support for the construct validity of the G-MAP measures.

Finally, the findings showed that different types of gamblers had different scores on the G-MAP measures, thus providing support for the criterion-related validity of the measures. In short, there is support for the different aspects of the validity of the G-MAP. Given the small sample size in the total sample and the problem gambler sample, the present findings can be regarded as robust and encouraging. In view of the paucity of psychosocial assessment tools in the Chinese context for problem gambling, this study is an important addition to the literature (16,17).

Table 6. Differences between problem gamblers and pathological gamblers on the G-MAP measures

Measures	Problem Gamblers		Pathological Gamblers		t value	
	Mean	S.D.	Mean	S.D.		
Control Scale	7.13	5.84	10.52	5.64	-1.65	*
Prophecy Scale	8.38	4.03	10.51	4.31	-1.37	ns
Uniformed Scale	8.25	4.13	14.54	4.37	-3.96	***
Good Feelings	6.38	4.98	9.83	5.01	-1.89	*
Boredom	6.88	4.97	10.76	5.32	-2.01	*
Numbness	9.00	4.28	8.28	4.27	.46	ns
Relaxation	5.75	4.13	10.02	4.88	-2.41	**
Desperation	3.25	3.49	8.80	4.91	-3.14	**
Transition Scale	4.25	6.07	8.37	5.50	-2.04	*
Oasis Scale	3.88	4.09	7.35	4.65	-2.06	*
Mischief Scale	4.50	4.41	6.03	4.60	-.92	ns
Negative Life-script Scale	5.75	3.85	9.66	5.36	-2.02	*
Entrenchment	11.25	4.50	12.94	3.44	-1.32	ns
Self Harm	5.63	5.80	4.02	3.81	1.11	ns
Winner Life-Script Scale	5.50	4.00	9.32	4.75	-2.22	*
Friendship Scale	2.00	1.85	5.98	4.15	-2.69	**
Shyness Scale	4.88	4.82	8.43	4.39	-2.21	*
Belief about Winning Domain	23.75	6.84	35.58	10.94	-3.01	**
Feelings Domain	28.00	16.13	38.89	15.67	-1.90	*
Situations Domain	15.88	13.64	30.55	15.92	-2.55	**
Attitudes to Self Domain	28.13	9.52	35.94	12.76	-1.70	*
Social Domain	6.88	5.79	14.42	7.92	-2.65	**
G-MAP	102.63	43.54	155.77	52.73	-2.79	**

* $p < .05$ (one-tailed).
** $p < .01$ (one-tailed).
*** $p < .001$ (one-tailed).
ns non-significant.

This work is also important in view of the growing addiction culture in Hong Kong (18) and there is a call for evidence-based welfare services in Hong Kong (19) and elsewhere (20).

Although our study provided some support for the reliability and validity of the Chinese G-MAP measures, further information should be collected for the test-retest reliability of the measures. Furthermore, additional studies on the convergent and discriminant validities of the Chinese G-MAP measures should be conducted in future. Finally, data collected from community samples would also substantiate the research and clinical utility of the G-MAP in the Chinese culture.

REFERENCES

[1] Petry NM. Pathological gambling: etiology, comorbidity, and treatment. Washington, DC: American Psychological Association, 2005.

[2] Cox BJ, Yu N, Afifi TO, Ladouceur R. A national survey of gambling problems in Canada. Can J Psychiatry 2005;50:213-7.

[3] Becona E. The prevalence of pathological gambling in Galicia according to the NODS. Reduction in prevalence or better assessment of the disorder? Adicciones 2004;16:173-84.
[4] Abbott MW, Volberg RA, Ronnberg S. Comparing the New Zealand and Swedish national surveys of gambling and problem gambling. J Gambl Stud 2004;20:237-58.
[5] General Education Centre of The Hong Kong Polytechnic University. Report on a study of Hong Kong people's participation in gambling activities. Hong Kong: General Education Centre, 2002.
[6] Fong DKC, Ozorio B. Gambling participation and prevalence estimates of pathological gambling in a far-east gambling city: Macao. UNLV Gambl Res Rev J 2005;9:15-28.
[7] Gupta R, Derevensky JL. Adolescent gambling behavior: a prevalence study and examination of the correlates associated with problem gambling. J Gambl Stud 1998;14:319-45.
[8] Gupta R, Derevensky JL. An examination of the differential coping style of adolescents with gambling problems. Montreal, Quebec: International Centre Youth Gambling Problems High-Risk Behavior, 2001.
[9] Langhinrichsen-Rohling J, Rohde P, Seeley JR, Rohling ML. Individual, family, peer correlates of adolescent gambling. J Gambl Stud 2004;20:23-46.
[10] Dickson LM, Derevensky JL, Gupta R. The prevention of gambling problems in youth: a conceptual framework. J Gambl Stud 2002;18:97-159.
[11] Hardoon KK, Gupta R, Derevensky JL. Psychosocial variables associated with adolescent gambling. Psychol Addict Behav 2004;18:170-9.
[12] Gupta R, Derevensky J. Adolescents with gambling problems: from research to treatment. J Gambl Stud 2000;16:315-42.
[13] Loughnan T, Pierce M, Sagris-Desmond A. Maroondah assessment profile for problem gambling: Administrator's manual. Melbourne: Australian Council Educational Research, 1999.
[14] American Psychiatric Association. Diagnostic and statistical manual of mental disorders: DSM-IV. Washington, DC: American Psychiatric Association, 1994.
[15] Schmitt N. Uses and abuses of coefficient alpha. Psychol Assess 1996;8:350-3.
[16] Shek DTL, ed. Research on social work practice in Chinese communities. Res Soc Work Pract 2002;12:485-581.
[17] Shek DTL, Chan YK, Lee P, eds. Special Issue on quality of life research in Chinese, Western and global contexts. Soc Indic Res 2005;71(1-3):1-539.
[18] Shek DTL. Tackling adolescent substance abuse in Hong Kong: where we should and should not go. ScientificWorldJournal 2007;7:2021–30.
[19] Shek DTL. Enthusiasm-based or evidence-based charities: personal reflections based on the Project P.A.T.H.S. in Hong Kong. ScientificWorldJournal 2008;8:802–10.
[20] Derevensky JL, Shek DTL, Merrick J, eds. Youth gambling. The hidden addiction. Berlin, De Gruyter, 2011.

In: Adolescence and Behavior Issues in a Chinese Context ISBN: 978-1-62618-614-9
Editors: DTL Shek, RCF Sun and Joav Merrick

Chapter 10

INTERNET ADDICTION IN CHINESE ADOLESCENTS IN HONG KONG: ASSESSMENT, PROFILES AND PSYCHOSOCIAL CORRELATES

Daniel TL Shek, PhD, FHKPS, BBS, JP [*1-5]
and Rachel CF Sun, PhD [6]
[1]Department of Applied Social Sciences,
The Hong Kong Polytechnic University, Hong Kong, PRC
[2] Centre for Innovative Programmes for Adolescents and Families,
The Hong Kong Polytechnic University, Hong Kong, PRC
[3]Department of Social Work, East China Normal University,
Shanghai, PRC
[4]Kiang Wu Nursing College of Macau, Macau, PRC
[5]Division of Adolescent Medicine, Department of Pediatrics,
Kentucky Children's Hospital,
University of Kentucky College of Medicine, Lexington, KY, US
[6]Faculty of Education, The University of Hong Kong, Hong Kong, PRC

ABSTRACT

Internet addiction behavior was examined in 6,121 Chinese primary and secondary school students in Hong Kong based on the assessment frameworks of Ivan Goldberg and Kimberly Young. Result showed that scales derived from both frameworks (CIA-Young Scale and CIA-Goldberg Scale) were internally consistent and evidence supporting their validity was found. Descriptive statistical analyses revealed that roughly one-fifth of the respondents could be classified as Internet addicted based on either scale. Further analyses showed that Internet addicted and non-addicted respondents differed in the Internet use and related behavior. Logistic regression analyses showed that engagement

[*] Correspondence: Professor Daniel T.L. Shek, PhD, FHKPS, BBS, JP, Chair Professor of Applied Social Sciences, Faculty of Health and Social Sciences, Department of Applied Social Sciences, The Hong Kong Polytechnic University, Room HJ407, Core H, Hunghom, Hong Kong. E-mail: daniel.shek@polyu.edu.hk.

in certain on-line activities (such as playing on-line games and downloading software) and replacement of pastimes activities (such as watching TV and going out with friends) by Internet activities predicted higher probability of Internet addiction.

INTRODUCTION

The Internet has become a basic tool for trading, entertainment, communication, as well as education in the contemporary world. Nevertheless, despite its positive uses, the presence of additive behaviors among some Internet users has drawn the attention of the public and helping professionals. In 1995, Ivan Goldberg borrowed criteria for defining psychoactive substance dependence in the DSM-IV and coined the term "Internet Addiction Disorder" to represent those having problematic Internet use behavior (1). Since then, a lot of research and debates about Internet addiction have been generated.

Similarly, as a leading expert in the field of problematic Internet use behavior, Kimberly Young developed the 7-item, 8-item, 10-item, and 20-item scales for assessing "Internet dependent" or "Internet addicted" behavior (2,3,4,5). In one of her study with a sample of 596 Internet users (1), Young found that 66% of the respondents could be classified as "Internet dependent", with the addictive behaviors including tolerance, loss of control, withdrawal, and impairment of functioning, which caused negative academic, social, financial, and occupational consequences (2).

There are other attempts to construct Internet addiction measurements. For example, Brenner developed a 32-item questionnaire entitled "Internet-Related Addictive Behavior Inventory" (IRABI) to assess Internet addiction and found that most of the respondents experienced at least one of the Internet addiction symptoms, including tolerance, craving, and withdrawal (1). Egger and Rauterberg (6) also designed a questionnaire to examine Internet behaviors and addiction tendency of 454 Internet users in Switzerland and other countries, and reported that 10.6% of the respondents were addicted to or dependent on the Internet.

Studies about Internet addiction have also been conducted in Chinese communities. In a study of 910 Taiwan college students, Chou and Hsiao (7) used the 40-item Chinese Internet-Related Addictive Behavior Inventory version II (C-IRABI-II) and Young's 8-item questionnaire to examine Internet addiction among the respondents. They found that 5.9% of the respondents could be classified as addicted to the Internet.

In another study of 2,203 adolescents from Taiwan, Ng, Choi, Cheung and Tsoi (8) adopted the 26-item Chinese Internet Addiction Scale and found that 10.7% of the respondents could be regarded as potentially at risk of Internet addiction, while 3.5% could be identified as seriously at risk of Internet addiction. In a study of 293 respondents from Fuzhou in mainland China, Lin and Yan (9) used the modified Young's 10-item questionnaire which showed that 9.6% of the respondents could be regarded as addicted to the Internet.

In Hong Kong, utilizing the Young's 20-item questionnaire to examine Internet addiction among 976 students, Tsuen Wan Centre of the Chinese YMCA of Hong Kong (10) found that 61.4% of senior primary school students, 35.2% of Secondary 1 to Secondary 3 students, 18.8% of Secondary 4 to Secondary 5 students, 35.8% of Secondary 6 to Secondary 7 students, and 37.0% of college students could be identified as highly at risk of Internet addiction. By comparing the data derived from two studies using the Young's 8-item questionnaire, Chan (11) found that the prevalence of Internet addiction had increased from

3.0% in 2000 to 14.7% in 2002. In another study of 1,182 adolescents, Yip and Kwok (12) used the modified Young's 8-item questionnaire which showed that 5.4% of the respondents as on-line game addicts.

There are also research findings showing that adolescents experienced the negative impact of Internet addictive behaviors. For example, in a study of 1,716 Secondary 1 to Secondary 3 students, Against Child Abuse (13) found that 37% of the respondents admitted that they "could not resist the attraction from being online" and 28.5% of the respondents agreed that "online activities largely affected their normal daily lives". Similarly, in a study of 677 pairs of parent-child, Choi, Wu, Zah and Ying (14) found that 14.5% of the parent respondents often had conflicts with their children regarding on-line problem. Regarding school performance, it was found that Internet addicted college students rated the impact of Internet on their study to be more negative than did their non-addicted counterparts (7). Parents also thought that there was negative impact on the academic performance of their children if they spent over 4.15 hours on the Internet daily (15). Finally, regarding the impact on psychosocial well-being, Internet addiction was found to be associated with subjective distress and social impairment (16).

Pratarelli, Browne and Johnson (17) argued that increased Internet use was associated with the feelings of isolation which were mutually reinforcing. Choi, Wu, Zah and Ying (14) also found that 17.1% of the adolescent respondents who spent more than 6 hours on-line daily had difficulty in controlling their unstable emotion.

There are several limitations pertinent to the existing literature on Internet addiction problem among adolescents in Chinese societies. First, few validated instruments are available and not many attempts have been made to develop and validate the assessment tools for Internet addiction.

Obviously, without valid and reliable assessment tools, it is difficult for helping professionals to identify adolescents with Internet addiction problem and develop intervention models to help them. Second, because most of the available studies were based on small samples, our understanding of Internet addiction problems among Chinese adolescents remains limited. Third, only few studies have examined the relationship between Internet use behavior (e.g., playing online games) and Internet addiction.

Against the above background, Internet addiction among primary and secondary school students was examined in this study using assessment tools based on the frameworks of Ivan Goldberg and Kimberly Young in Chinese context (i.e., CIA-Goldberg scale and CIA-Young Scale). Several research questions are addressed in this paper: 1) What are the psychometric properties of the CIA-Goldberg Scale and CIA-Young Scale? 2) What are the profiles of responses to the items in the CIA-Goldberg Scale and CIA-Young Scale? 3) What are the differences between Internet addicted and non-addicted adolescents in terms of Internet use and related behavior? 4) What factors predict Internet addiction in young people in Hong Kong?

The findings reported in this paper were based on a project entitled "Youngster Internet Addiction Prevention and Counseling Service" funded by the Community Chest of Hong Kong, which was aimed at providing preventive and counseling services for young people displaying Internet addiction problem.

OUR STUDY

A convenient sample with 6,121 students recruited from 16 primary and secondary schools in Hong Kong was used. Most of the respondents were aged between 11 to 18 years (97.7%). The three dominant age groups in the sample included the 15-16 years group (25.5%), 13-14 years group (37.6%) and 11-12 years group (21.8%). There were slightly more males (51.2%) than females (48.8%) in the sample. Regarding the duration that the participants had been using the Internet, 18.6% had used for 3.0 to 3.9 years, 17.2% had used for 4.0 to 4.9 years, 20% had used for 5.0-5.9 years, and less than 5% of the sample had been using the Internet for 8 years or above at the time of the study. Each respondent was invited to complete a self-administered questionnaire that contained different measures of Internet addiction symptoms, Internet usage, and background information (e.g., family income, academic performance and conduct at school, perceived quality of family life). The questionnaire is available upon request from the first author.

To give a comprehensive assessment of Internet addiction, two measures were used in this study. These included:

- The Chinese Internet Addiction (Goldberg) Scale (CIA-Goldberg). In 1995, Ivan Goldberg borrowed the criteria of substance abuse in the DSM-IV and proposed seven criteria to assess whether a person can be defined as having "Internet Addiction Disorder" (18). A person who meets three or more criteria is defined as having "Internet Addiction Disorder". The first and second authors translated the criteria into Chinese.
- The Chinese Internet Addiction (Young) Scale (CIA-Young). Kimberly Young developed several versions of assessment tools, including Young's 7-item questionnaire, Young's brief 8-item questionnaire, and Young's 10-item questionnaire. The items in the first and second assessment tools were developed with reference to the criteria for pathological gambling in the DSM-IV and psychoactive substance dependence in the DSM-IV, respectively (2,4). Young's 10-item questionnaire (3) was employed in this study. A person who answers "Yes" to four or more of the questions is defined as "Internet dependent". The items were translated by the first and second authors.

Based on a review of the existing literature in both Western and Chinese communities (6,17,19), 13 items were developed by the first and second authors to understand the frequency of using the Internet and activities engaged (e.g., playing on-line games, downloading software, meeting new friends) in the last twelve months among the respondents. In addition, two Internet addiction/dependence questions based on self-assessment were developed: "Do you consider yourself to be addicted to the Internet?" and "Do you consider yourself excessively use or depend on the Internet to satisfy different kinds of need?" The respondents gave their answers on a 5-point scale (1 =definitely not to 5= absolutely yes).

The data for our study were collected in the context of school talks. After the third author of the present study and/or his colleagues obtained consent of the 16 schools, data were collected from students before the school talk on the topic related to healthy Internet usage which was delivered by a social worker in each school. The purpose of the study was mentioned and the confidentiality of data collected was repeatedly emphasized to all of the students in attendance on the day of testing. The students participated in the study on a voluntary basis. They were asked to indicate their wish if they did not want to participate in the study (i.e., 'passive' informed consent was obtained from the students).

At least one school staff (with most of them were teachers) was present throughout the test administration session. Adequate time was provided for the respondents to complete the questionnaire in self-report format. The respondents generally took 20 to 30 minutes to complete the questionnaire.

OUR FINDINGS

Psychometric properties of CIA-Goldberg and CIA-Young

Results showed that the internal consistency of CIA-Goldberg and CIA-Young was good. Cronbach's alpha for CIA-Goldberg and CIA-Young was .68 and .75 respectively. Regarding validity of the scales, findings based on Pearson correlation analyses showed that both scales were moderately related to whether one was self-assessed as Internet addict and whether there was excessively usage of or dependence on Internet.

The scale scores were also significantly related to the time spent on Internet activities (Table 1).

Table 1. Relationships between two assessment tools of Internet addiction (CIA-Goldberg and CIA-Young) and other measures of excessive Internet use

	Self-assessed as addicted to the Internet	Self-assessed as excessively use or depend on the Internet	Average amount of total Internet time per week	Average amount of Internet time spend on entertainment per week
CIA-Goldberg	.406*	.393*	.188*	.186*
CIA-Young	.423*	.412*	.216*	.207*

* $p < 0.001$ (Bonferroni-corrected alpha level = 0.006).

Profiles of responses to the CIA-Goldberg and CIA-Young

The percentages of responses to the questions in CIA-Goldberg and CIA-Young are presented in Table 2 and Table 3, respectively. Using the cutoff score of 3, 22.9% (N =1,371) of the respondents could be classified as Internet addicted using the CIA-Goldberg. On the other hand, 19.1% (N =1,150) of the respondents could be identified as Internet addicted based on the CIA-Young.

Table 2. Percentages of responses to the questions in CIA-Goldberg

Criterion	Question	*N*	%	
			Yes	No
1	(a) Do you find there is a diminished effect with continued use of the same time spent on the Internet?	6106	13.3xxx	86.7
	(b) Do you experience a tolerance in that you have a need for increased amounts of Internet use to achieve the desired effect?	6121	21.9	78.1
2	Do you access Internet more often or for longer periods of time than you intended?	6102	32.2	67.8
3	Have you had a persistent desire or made unsuccessful efforts to cut down or control the amount of time spend online?	6081	16.4	83.6
4	Do you spend a great deal of time in activities related to Internet use (e.g., buying Internet books, trying out new WWW browsers, organizing files of downloaded materials)?	6102	26.6	73.4
5	Have you given up or reduced any important social, occupational, academic or recreational activities because of the Internet use?	6099	18.0	82.0
6	Have you continued to use the Internet despite knowledge of having physical, social, occupational, academic or psychological problem (e.g., sleep deprivation, interpersonal conflicts, lateness for work, lateness for school, neglect of student or occupational duties)?	6102	18.1	81.9
7	(a) Have you made attempts to cut down the excessive amount of time you spend on-line? (b) Have the following condition been developed within several days to a month after you made attempts to cut down the excessive amount of time you spend on-line?	5942	42.4	57.6

Criterion	Question		*N*	%	
				Yes	No
	I	I have had psychomotor agitation.	5751	6.0	94.0
	II	I have felt anxious.	5751	3.0	97.0
	III	I have had obsessive thinking about what is happening on Internet	5751	9.9	90.1
	IV	I have had fantasies or dreams about Internet.	5751	6.0	94.0
	V	My fingers have done typing movements voluntarily or involuntarily.	5751	2.1	97.9
	(c) Have you used the Internet as a way of relieving or avoiding the above unwell condition?		5745	4.8	95.2
	(d) Do you feel that the above condition cause distress or impairment in your social, occupational or another important area of functioning?		5718	4.3	95.7
Overall "Internet Addicted" Percentage (met 3 or more criteria)			6000	**22.9**	77.1

Table 3. Percentages of responses to the questions in CIA-Young

	Question	*N*	%	
			Yes	No
1	Do you feel preoccupied with the Internet or on-line services and think about it while off-line?	6118	25.2	74.8
2	Do you feel a need to spend more and more time on-line to achieve satisfaction?	6121	21.9	78.1
3	Have you repeatedly made unsuccessful efforts to control, cut back, or stop Internet use?	6104	17.6	82.4
4	Do you feel restless, moody, depressed, or irritable when attempting to cut down or stop Internet use?	6106	12.3	87.7
5	Do you stay on-line longer than original intended?	6118	41.4	58.6
6	Have you jeopardized or risked the loss of significant relationship, job, educational or career opportunity because of the Internet?	6114	22.5	77.5
7	Have you lied to family members, teachers, social workers, or others to conceal the extent of involvement with the Internet?	6102	11.3	88.7
8	Do you use the Internet as a way of escaping from problems or of relieving a dysphoric mood (e.g., feelings of helplessness, guilt, anxiety, depression)?	6105	12.0	88.0
9	Do you keep returning even after spending too much money on on-line fees?	6103	15.9	84.1
10	Do you feel depressed, irritable, moody or anxious when you are off-line?	6114	11.2	88.8
Overall "Internet Addicted" Percentage (answered "Yes" to 4 or more questions)		6024	**19.1**	80.9

Table 4. Comparison of Internet usage between Internet Addicted (IA) and Non-Internet Addicted (NIA) respondents

		Mean			
		Tool 1 (C-Goldberg)		Tool 2 (C-Young)	
		IA	NIA	IA	NIA
1	Average amount of Internet time spend on entertainment per week (in hours)	15.8	9.1***	17.1	9.1***
2	Average amount of Internet time spend on study per week (in hours)	3.1	2.7	3.3	2.7*
3	Average amount of total Internet time per week (in hours)	17.7	10.5***	19.5	10.5***
4	Number of new acquaintances have made solely on the Internet	14.4	8.3	16.7	8.5*
5	Number of clubs or organizations belong to on the Internet	6.8	2.8**	7.1	2.9**
6	Frequency of engaging in the following Internet activities (answered 1= *never* to 4= *very often*)				
	I Playing On-line games	3.18	2.70***	3.20	2.72***
	II Downloading software	2.97	2.49***	2.94	2.52***
	III Talking to friends who immigrate to or study at overseas (e.g., chat room, ICQ)	2.75	2.43***	2.75	2.45***
	IV Keeping track of new developments in the areas of personal interest (e.g., computer accessories, football, beauty, on-line games)	3.05	2.69***	3.01	2.71***
	V Downloading information (e.g., songs, movies, mobile phone ring tones)	3.16	2.68***	3.13	2.71***
	VI Reading and posting message on newsgroup / discussion group	2.49	2.15***	2.48	2.16***
	VII Meeting new friends	2.37	1.92***	2.45	1.92***
	VIII Updating personal homepage	2.05	1.78***	2.07	1.80***
	IX Seeking advices on different areas of life (e.g., interpersonal relationship, health) from professionals	1.94	1.76***	1.97	1.76***
	X Talking to on-line friends who share my interests	3.05	2.52***	3.07	2.54***
	XI WWW-surfing, browsing	3.34	3.11***	3.29	3.13***

Table 4. (Continued)

			Mean			
			Tool 1 (C-Goldberg)		Tool 2 (C-Young)	
			IA	NIA	IA	NIA
7	Level of Internet replacing the following activities or pastimes (answered 1= *never* to 4= *very often*)					
	I	Watching TV	2.98	2.73***	2.99	2.74***
	II	Talking to friends in person	2.49	2.28***	2.50	2.29***
	III	Going out with family	2.32	2.17***	2.37	2.16***
	IV	Participating in activities inside or outside school	2.21	2.06***	2.20	2.07***
	V	Going out with friends	2.48	2.20***	2.50	2.20***

*** $p < 0.001$.

** $p < 0.005$.

* $p < 0.05$.

Table 5. Logistic regression of activities engaged online and activities or pastimes replaced by Internet based on Tool 1 (CIA-Goldberg)

Variables in the Equation	B	S.E.	Wald	df	Sig.	Exp(B)
Internet related activities						
Searching information for school related assignments	-.282	.048	34.176	1	.000	.754
Reading and writing e-mails	-.119	.042	7.875	1	.005	.888
Playing On-line games	.345	.040	74.068	1	.000	1.412
Downloading software	.254	.045	31.830	1	.000	1.289
Talking to friends at overseas	-.022	.037	.353	1	.552	.979
Keeping track of new developments in the areas of personal interest	.147	.042	12.572	1	.000	1.159
Downloading information	.142	.041	12.226	1	.000	1.153
Reading and posting message on newsgroup / discussion group	.064	.038	2.757	1	.097	1.066
Meeting new friends	.149	.041	13.409	1	.000	1.161
Updating personal homepage	.087	.037	5.553	1	.018	1.091
Seeking advices from professionals	.029	.046	.397	1	.529	1.029
Talking to on-line friends	.164	.039	17.441	1	.000	1.178
WWW-surfing, browsing	.059	.046	1.619	1	.203	1.061
Replacement of leisure time activities by Internet activities						
Watching TV replaced by Internet	.192	.037	26.345	1	.000	1.212
Talking to friends in person replaced by Internet	.056	.040	1.937	1	.164	1.058
Going out with family replaced by Internet	.021	.041	.273	1	.601	1.022
Participating in activities inside or outside school replaced by Internet	-.015	.037	.163	1	.686	.985
Going out with friends replaced by Internet	.141	.037	14.456	1	.000	1.151

Table 6. Logistic regression of activities engaged online and activities or pastimes replaced by Internet based on Tool 2 (CIA-Young)

Variables in the Equation	B	S.E.	Wald	df	Sig.	Exp(B)
Internet related activities						
Searching information for school related assignments	-.380	.051	54.760	1	.000	.684
Reading and writing e-mails	-.096	.045	4.554	1	.033	.908
Playing On-line games	.355	.043	67.498	1	.000	1.426
Downloading software	.193	.048	16.244	1	.000	1.213
Talking to friends at overseas	-.020	.039	.274	1	.601	.980
Keeping track of new developments in the areas of personal interest	.123	.044	7.679	1	.006	1.131
Downloading information	.079	.043	3.291	1	.070	1.082
Reading and posting message on newsgroup / discussion group	.060	.041	2.176	1	.140	1.062
Meeting new friends	.259	.043	36.930	1	.000	1.296
Updating personal homepage	.094	.039	5.800	1	.016	1.099
Seeking advices from professionals	.080	.048	2.730	1	.099	1.083
Talking to on-line friends	.162	.043	14.443	1	.000	1.176
WWW-surfing, browsing	-.019	.049	.148	1	.700	.981
Replacement of leisure time activities by Internet activities						
Watching TV replaced by Internet	.171	.040	18.306	1	.000	1.187
Talking to friends in person replaced by Internet	.034	.043	.633	1	.426	1.035
Going out with family replaced by Internet	.108	.043	6.263	1	.012	1.114
Participating in activities inside or outside school replaced by Internet	-.075	.040	3.589	1	.058	.927
Going out with friends replaced by Internet	.171	.039	18.732	1	.000	1.186

Differences between Internet addicted and non-addicted respondents

Results showed that the Internet-addicted and non-addicted groups could be differentiated in terms the related scale scores (Table 4). Using CIA-Goldberg, the addicted group displayed a higher score than did the non-addicted group (mean = 3.896 and 0.689 for the Addicted Group and Non-Addicted Group, respectively; $t = 101.754$, $p < .001$; Cohen's $d = 0.95$). Using CIA-Young, the addicted group displayed a higher score than did the non-addicted group (mean = 5.511 and 1.061 for the Addicted Group and Non-Addicted Group, respectively; $t = 86.997$, $p < .001$; Cohen's $d = 1.39$).

Results further showed several phenomena: a) Internet addicted respondents spent more time online than their non-addicted counterparts; b) the Internet addicted respondents made more new acquaintances solely on the Internet than their non-addicted counterparts; c) the Internet addicted respondents belonged to more clubs or organizations on the Internet than their non-addicted counterparts; d) the Internet addicted respondents engaged in various kinds of Internet activity more frequent than their non-addicted counterparts; e) Internet addicted respondents had a stronger tendency to replace different kinds of offline activity or pastime than their non-addicted counterparts.

Predictors of Internet addiction

Logistic regression analyses consistently showed that several predictors increased the likelihood of being classified as Internet addicted (Table 5 and Table 6). These factors included certain on-line activities (such as playing on-line games, downloading software and meeting new friend) and replacement of leisure time activities by Internet activities.

DISCUSSION

Research findings varied a lot on the rates of Internet addition among youth, probably because different questionnaires were used. Despite different questionnaires for assessing Internet addition were developed, tolerance, withdrawal, and impairment of psychosocial functioning were often included. However, some researchers argued that it was not appropriate to define Internet addiction as a unique psychiatric disorder as the validity of the construct was doubtful. For instance, the existence of wide range of Internet activities suggested that Internet addiction was unlikely to be a single phenomenon. Besides, the question about co-morbidity conditions suggested that Internet addiction might just be an expression of other disorders (20). Grohol (21) argued that people would go from overuse to balance eventually, while the overuse was only a transition phase. These arguments suggest that reliable and valid assessment tools that can capture the dynamic nature of Internet addiction are badly needed.

In addition, many researchers about Internet addiction collected their data through Internet surveys, such as e-mail surveying and World Wide Web (WWW) surveying, which led to the problems of sampling bias. For instance, in a review of Internet-based survey research, Brenner (22) pointed out that one significant bias of Internet addiction surveys was the over representation of the male respondents.

Besides, the small sample size of the available studies was another issue – there were 76 respondents in Li and Chung's (23) study, 100 respondents in Nalwa and Anand's (24) study, and 271 respondents in Wang's (25) study. All these observations call for the need for developing reliable and valid Internet addiction measures through careful research designs.

In this study, the psychometric properties of two developed measures of Internet addiction were examined through 6,121 students, with similar proportions of male and female respondents. Results showed that the CIA-Goldberg and CIA-Young were internally consistent. In addition, the evidence for the construct validity of the two developed measures of Internet addiction were found, including the positive relationships between CIA-Goldberg and CIA-Young and measures of: a) self-assessment of Internet addiction, b) self-assessment of excessive use of or dependence on the Internet, c) amount of time spend on Internet, and d) amount of Internet time spent on entertainment. With reference to the concern of lacking reliable and valid assessment tools for Internet addiction, the present study is a significant addition to the Chinese literature on Internet addiction among young people.

Based on the CIA-Goldberg and CIA-Young, 22.9% and 19.1% of the respondents in this study could be identified as Internet addicted, which were similar to the results found in some of the existing studies targeting on adolescents (26,27). As Internet addiction adversely affected one's physical health, family life and academic performance (28) and caused severe psychological distress (29), the present findings alert us the need for early identification of adolescents having Internet addiction and high risk for Internet addiction.

Several differences were found between the respondents in the Internet-addicted and non-addicted groups identified by CIA-Goldberg and CIA-Young in this study. First, the Internet addicted respondents spent more time online than the non-addicted, which is consistent with the findings of previous studies (30,31). Second, the Internet addicted respondents made more new acquaintances on the Internet, a finding which is consistent with the result shown in Egger and Rauterberg's study (6). Third, the Internet addicted respondents belonged to more clubs or organizations on the Internet than the non-addicted, a finding which echoes the result shown in the study of Whang, Lee and Chang (32). Fourth, consistent with the previous findings (7,33), the Internet addicted respondents engaged in various kinds of Internet activity more frequent than the non-addicted.

Based on the two measurements of Internet addiction in this study, it was found that the frequency of engaging in on-line activities, including playing on-line games, downloading software, meeting new friends and talking to on-line friends, were powerful predictors of Internet addiction. Besides, the frequency of leisure time activities, including watching TV and going out with friends replaced by Internet activities, were also powerful in predicting Internet addiction.

In other words, the more frequent one engages in the above mentioned on-line activities and replaces TV-watching and going out with friends by Internet activities, the more likely he or she will be addicted to the Internet. As there are few research studies examining the predictors of Internet addiction in Chinese adolescents, the present findings can be regarded as pioneering additions to the literature.

It is noteworthy that there are several limitations of the present study. First, as a convenient sample was used, generalizability of the present findings to the population should be addressed with caution. Second, the findings should be interpreted with reference to the debates surrounding to the validity of the construct of Internet addiction. Third, if resource permits, Internet addiction based on ratings by psychiatrists should be added to further assess the criterion-related validity of the developed tools.

Finally, as the significant correlation among the variables may be due to common method variance, further work utilizing multitrait-multimethod strategy should be carried out. Despite these limitations, the present findings provide some pioneering findings on Internet addiction among Chinese adolescents in Hong Kong.

ACKNOWLEDGMENT

The Youngster Internet Addiction Prevention and Counseling Service undertaken by the Jockey Club Wah Ming Lutheran Integrated Service Centre, Hong Kong Lutheran Social Service, LC-HKS was funded by the Community Chest of Hong Kong. Preparation for this paper was financially supported by the Wofoo Foundation Limited.

REFERENCES

[1] Danforth IDW. Addiction to online game: classification and personality correlates. [monograph on the Internet]. Accessed 2012 Sep 7. URL: http://www.iandanforth.net/pdfs/addiction.pdf

[2] Griffiths M. Internet addiction: does it really exist? In: Gackenbach J, ed. Psychology and the Internet: intrapersonal, interpersonal, and transpersonal implications. San Diego, CA: Academic Press, 1998:61-75.

[3] Suler J. Computer and cyberspace addiction. Int J Applied Psychoanal Studies 2004;1:359-62.

[4] Young KS. Caught in the net: how to recognize the signs of Internet addiction and a winning strategy of recovery. New York: Wiley, 1998.

[5] Young KS. A therapist's guide to assess and treat Internet addiction: a exclusive guide for practitioners. [monograph on the Internet]. 1999 Accessed 2012 Sep 7. URL: http://www.netaddiction.com/downloads.html

[6] Egger O, Rauterberg M. Internet behavior and addiction. [monograph on the Internet]. Zurich: Work & Organizational Psychology Unit (IfAP), Swiss Federal Institute of Technology; 1996. Accessed 2012 Sep 7. URL: http://www.ipo.tue.nl/homepages/mrauterb/publications/INTERNET96report.pdf

[7] Chou C, Hsiao MC. Internet addiction, usage, gratification, and pleasure experience: the Taiwan college students' case. Computers Educ 2000;35:65-80.

[8] Ng SH, Choi LM, Cheung SW, Tsoi TY. Internet addiction and bullying of Taipei's adolescent. [monograph on the Internet]. PRC: Taipei Adolescent Counseling Committee, 2003. Accessed 2012 Sep 7. URL: http://jcc.tmpd.gov.tw/%BA%F4%B8%F4%B3Q%AE.pdf

[9] Lin XH, Yan GG. Internet addiction disorder, online behavior and personality. Chinese Mental Health J 2001;15(4):281-3.

[10] Tsuen Wan Centre, Chinese YMCA of Hong Kong. Study on adolescents' Internet using behaviors. Hong Kong: Tsuen Wan Centre, Chinese YMCA of Hong Kong, 2004.

[11] Chan TCF. Cyberrisk of Hong Kong Youngsters. J Youth Studies 2004; 7(2 Serial 14):155-68.

[12] Yip WS, Kwok YK. Adolescents' computer using phenomena. Hong Kong: Hong Kong Christian Service, 2005.

[13] Against Child Abuse. The impacts of Internet on junior secondary school students: a research report. Hong Kong: Against Child Abuse, 2004.

[14] Choi, CW, Wu KT, Zah KK, Ying CW. The impacts of Internet on adolescents' family relationships and mental health: a research report. Hong Kong: Hong Kong Family Welfare Society, 2005.

[15] Cheng HCH, Chan YC. Parental perception on children's Internet use: a research report. Hong Kong: Centre for Social Policy Studies, Department of Applied Social Sciences, Hong Kong Polytechnic University, Tung Wah Group of Hospitals, 2004.
[16] Shapira NA, Goldsmith TD, Keck Jr PE, Khosla UM, McElroy, SL. Psychiatric features of individuals with problematic internet use. J Affect Disord 2000;57:267-72.
[17] Pratarelli ME, Browne BL, Johnson K. The bits and bytes of computer/Internet addiction: a factor analytic approach. Behav Res Methods Instruments Computers 1999;31(2):305-14.
[18] Suler J. Internet addiction support group: is there truth in jest? In: The Psychology of Cyberspace. [hypertext book on the Internet]. 1996. Accessed 2012 Sep 7. URL: http://www.rider.edu/~suler/psycyber/supportgp.html
[19] Commission on Youth. Study on the influence of information technology on youth. Hong Kong: Commission on Youth, 2001.
[20] Shaffer HJ, Hall MN, Bilt JV. Computer addiction: a critical consideration. Am J Orthopsy 2000;70(2):162-8.
[21] Grohol JM. Internet addiction guide. [monograph on the Internet]. 1999. Accessed 2012 Sep 7. URL: http://psychcentral.com/netaddiction
[22] Brenner V. Generalizability issues in Internet-based survey research: implications for the Internet addiction controversy. In: Batinic B, Reips U, Bosnjok M, eds. Online social sciences. Seattle: Hogrefe Huber, 2002: 93-144.
[23] Li SM, Chung TM. Internet function and Internet addictive behavior. Computers Hum Behav 2006;22:1067-71.
[24] Nalwa K, Anand AP. Internet addiction in students: a cause of concern. Cyber Psychol Behav 2003;6(6):653-6.
[25] Wang W. Internet dependency and psychosocial maturity among college students. Int J Hum Computer Stud 2001;55:919-38.
[26] Johansson A, Götestam KG. Internet addiction: characteristic of a questionnaire and prevalence in Norwegian youth (12-18 years). Scand J Psychol 2004;45:223-9.
[27] Lee MS, Ko YH, Song HS, Kwon KH, Lee HS, Nam M, et al. Characteristics of Internet use in relation to game genre in Korean adolescents. Cyber Psychol Behav 2007;10(2):278-85.
[28] Young K. Internet addiction: symptoms, evaluation, and treatment. In: VandeCreek L, Jackson T, eds. Innovations in clinical practice: a source book vol.17. Sarasota, FL: Professional Resource Press, 1999:19-31.
[29] Hur MH. Demographic, habitual, and socioeconomic determinants of Internet addiction disorder: an empirical study of Korean teenagers. Cyber Psychol Behav 2006;9(5):514-25.
[30] Anderson KJ. Internet use among college students: an exploratory study. [book on the Internet]. Accessed 2012 Sep 7. URL: http://www.rpi.edu/~anderk4/research.html
[31] Yen JY, Ko CH, Yen CF, Wu HY, Yang MJ. The comorbid psychiatric symptoms of Internet addiction: attention deficit and hyperactivity disorder (ADHD), depression, social phobia and hostility. J Adolesc Health 2007;41:93-8.
[32] Whang LS, Lee S, Chang G. Internet over-users' psychological profiles: a behavior sampling analysis on Internet addiction. Cyber Psychol Behav 2003;6(2):143-50.
[33] Yuen CN, Lavin MJ. Internet dependence in the collegiate population: the role of shyness. Cyber Psychol Behav 2004;7(4):379-83.

In: Adolescence and Behavior Issues in a Chinese Context
Editors: DTL Shek, RCF Sun and Joav Merrick
ISBN: 978-1-62618-614-9

Chapter 11

FAMILY PROCESSES AND SUICIDAL IDEATION AMONG CHINESE ADOLESCENTS IN HONG KONG

***Sylvia YCL Kwok*[1] *and Daniel TL Shek*[2-6] ***

[1]Department of Applied Social Studies,
The City University of Hong Kong, Hong Kong, PRC
[2]Department of Applied Social Sciences,
The Hong Kong Polytechnic University, Hong Kong, PRC
[3]Public Policy Research Institute,
The Hong Kong Polytechnic University, Hong Kong, PRC
[4]Department of Social Work, East China Normal University,
Shanghai, PRC
[5]Kiang Wu Nursing College of Macau, Macau, PRC
[6]Division of Adolescent Medicine, Department of Pediatrics,
Kentucky Children's Hospital,
University of Kentucky College of Medicine, Lexington, KY, US

ABSTRACT

This chapter is based on the responses of 5,557 Chinese secondary students in Hong Kong, the relationships between perceived family functioning (systemic correlate), as well as parent-adolescent communication (dyadic correlate), and suicidal ideation. Results showed that suicidal ideation was negatively related to global family functioning and parent-adolescent communication. Regression analyses indicated that the dyadic and systemic factors had similar importance in predicting suicidal ideation. Theoretical and practical implications of the findings are discussed.

* Correspondence: Professor Daniel T.L. Shek, PhD, FHKPS, BBS, JP, Chair Professor of Applied Social Sciences, Faculty of Health and Social Sciences, Department of Applied Social Sciences, The Hong Kong Polytechnic University, Room HJ407, Core H, Hunghom, Hong Kong. E-mail: daniel.shek@polyu.edu.hk.

INTRODUCTION

A review of Confucianism, Buddhism and Taoism as major Chinese religions and philosophies shows that they are opposed to suicidal behaviors (1). In Confucian thinking, it is maintained that "body, hair and skin" come from parents, therefore one dares not to damage" (shen ti fa fu, shou zhu fu mu, bu gan hui shang). In Buddhism, the importance of "non-killing" (bu xia sheng) of living things (including oneself) is emphasized. Actually, "killing" is one of the acts that Buddhists should avoid as far as possible, while Taoists emphasize the heaven's virtue in preserving life (shun tian er xing).

Suicide statistics and related phenomena in Hong Kong and the United States

Despite these cultural influences, an examination of the suicide statistics indicates that suicide rates in Chinese people are not particularly low. For example, Shek, Lee and Chow (2) showed that suicide rates in rural China were high and suicide rates amongst young people in Hong Kong were gradually rising in the 1990s. Adolescent suicidal ideation is also an emerging social problem in Hong Kong in the recent years. In two studies of adolescents aged 12 to 18 with 2,427 and 1,309 subjects, 17.8% and 12.8% reported having suicidal ideation respectively (3,4). Even more disturbing, another study examining the predictors of suicidal ideation and depression in Hong Kong adolescents reported that 47% of 327 Chinese female students aged 13 to 18 (Study 1) and 52.6% of 371 Chinese adolescents aged 14 to 20 (Study 2) had experienced suicidal ideation (5). The rate of adolescent suicidal ideation in the United States is similar. For example, based on the National Youth Risk Behavior Survey conducted in 2005 in the United States, it was found that 16.9% of 13,953 grade 9 to grade 12 students from public and private schools, reported suicidal ideation (6). However, it is noteworthy that there are differences in the suicidal ideation scales used. As suicidal ideation is highly correlated with suicide attempts (7,8), more in-depth study of the correlates of suicidal ideation is essential.

There are studies in Hong Kong and the United States showing that family processes are related to adolescent suicidal ideation. In Hong Kong, different studies revealed that an uncaring family environment, negative family climate, low levels of family cohesion and support, high level of parent-adolescent conflict, parental rejection and over-control were associated with adolescent suicidal thoughts (5,9,10). Similarly, previous studies in the United States found that adolescent suicidal ideation was positively related to family dysfunction, family discord, poor family environment, family rigidity, family conflicts and poor adaptability, but negatively related to perceived parental support and family support (11,12,13).

Although similar research findings in the United States and Hong Kong are reported, there are two significant areas of difference. First, research findings show that Hong Kong adolescents are more dependent on their families for emotional and instrumental support than adolescents in the United States (14). As such, it is interesting to ask whether the influence of family processes on adolescent suicidal ideation would be different within Hong Kong. Second, as the subjects being studied are Chinese adolescents living in Hong Kong, they are under the strong influence of Chinese culture. Hong Kong is regarded as a Chinese society and the families in Hong Kong are usually referred to as Chinese families. Since Chinese families have some characteristics that are different from those of the Western ones, e.g. emphasis on harmony and non-expression of emotions (15), it would be interesting to study how family processes are related to adolescent suicidal ideation in Hong Kong families.

Gaps in the existing studies related to family processes and suicidal ideation

First, the existing findings on the relationship between family correlates and adolescent suicidal ideation are equivocal. For example, a study in the United States by Mitchell and Rosenthal (16) found no significant group difference in terms of the mean family rigidity scores in the families of suicidal and non-suicidal psychiatric inpatient adolescents. In addition, no association between perceived parent-adolescent relationship and adolescent suicidal behavior was found in another United States study (17).

Second, although there are differences in the cultural norms for "healthy" family functioning between Western and Chinese societies, there are very few studies utilizing indigenous Chinese measures of family functioning. According to a study on the attributes of happy families in Hong Kong (15,18), Chinese parents and their children regarded the absence of conflict, interpersonal harmony, mutuality, connectedness, and positive parent-adolescent relationships as important attributes of a happy family. Although contemporary Western societies emphasize mutual respect among family members, Chinese families are more hierarchical in structure (19,20). For example, Chinese wives are taught to be submissive to their husbands and children are socialized to obey their fathers, in accordance with the *wu lun* in traditional Chinese culture (21). In view of the difference between Western and Chinese culture, it would be theoretically important to ask whether the hypothesized negative relationship between family functioning and adolescent suicidal ideation can be found in the Chinese culture.

Third, few studies have been conducted to examine parent-adolescent communication and adolescent suicidal ideation both in the United States and Hong Kong (22,23) Even given the limited number of studies, there are inconsistent findings, particularly with respect to gender and parental differences in the linkage between parent-adolescent communication and suicidal ideation. For example, while Adams, Overholser and Lehnert (24) showed that perceived problems in communication with the mother but not with the father differentiated suicidal adolescents from nonsuicidal adolescents, King, Hill, Naylor, and Shain (25) showed that suicidal adolescents reported less active and communicative relationships with the fathers but not with the mothers in the United States. Basically, one should ask whether the linkages between these two domains are different in father-son, father-daughter, mother-son and mother-daughter dyads.

Studies in the United States and Hong Kong showed a stronger impact of parents on girls than on boys (26,27), while mother-adolescent relationship had a stronger impact on adolescent developmental outcomes than did father-adolescent relationship (28,29). Hence, whether mother-adolescent communication exerts a stronger influence on adolescent suicidal ideation than does father-adolescent communication should be examined.

Fourth, most of the measuring instruments on parent-adolescent communication for the Hong Kong studies were adapted from the West, which may not be able to capture the essence of the Chinese culture. In the traditional Chinese culture, open parent-adolescent communication was basically not encouraged because children were taught to inhibit their expression of feelings and exhibit a general pattern of respect, obedience and piety (30). Within such a cultural context, this repression of feelings and opinions should also be included in analyzing parent-adolescent communication process. Hence, one should develop indigenous measures of parent-adolescent communication to examine the related issues with reference to the uniqueness of the Chinese culture.

Fifth, it is not clear which family process, if any, is comparatively more important than others. Within the family system, three basic processes are present, including individual process (e.g. development of resilience), dyadic process (e.g. parent-adolescent communication) and systemic process (e.g. family functioning). Previous findings on their relative importance are equivocal. A study found that after controlling for other causal factors (e.g. family adaptability and cohesion), poorer parent-adolescent communication remained strongly associated with adolescent self-harm (31). On the contrary, another study showed that family strengths had an indirect effect on adolescent depression through self-esteem, while parent-adolescent communication did not have a direct effect or an indirect effect on adolescent depression (32). Although some studies stressed both parent-adolescent communication and family functioning as important predictors of adolescent suicidal ideation (33), it is theoretically important to ask whether systemic or dyadic mechanism is more important for predicting suicidal ideation. For example, as family communication involves interaction among different family members including grandparents and siblings while parent-adolescent communication includes only the parent-adolescent dyad, their effects on adolescent suicidal ideation may be different.

Conceptual framework

The family systems theory (34) is adopted in this study. As the family is a system composed of interconnected and interdependent individuals, a person cannot be understood in isolation from the family system. An individual's behavior is caused by interaction with other family members and dynamics within the family system as a whole. Hence, to understand adolescent suicidal ideation, it is important to examine the family processes that include the adolescents' interaction with the parents (i.e. dyadic process, parent-adolescent communication) and the impact of the family system (i.e. systemic process, family functioning) on their thinking and behaviors. The systems perspective has been used to look at the relationship among individual, dyadic and systemic processes in the family. For example, Shek (29) adopted the systems perspective to understand how individual and dyadic processes contribute to systemic family functioning. Based on the family systems perspective, a conceptual model was formulated and several research questions were addressed in this study (see figure 1).

The first research question is: what is the relationship between parent-adolescent communication and Chinese adolescent suicidal ideation in Hong Kong? Based on the family systems theory that child development is affected by interaction with their parents (34) and previous research findings (35), it was hypothesized that parent-adolescent communication would have a negative relationship with adolescent suicidal ideation (Hypothesis 1).

With reference to previous studies (26,28), it was hypothesized that mother-adolescent communication would have a more significant relationship than father-adolescent communication with suicidal ideation, especially for female adolescents (Hypothesis 1a).

Furthermore, as research findings showed that fathers exerted stronger influence on daughters than on sons, it would be expected that father-adolescent communication would have a stronger association with suicidal ideation in daughters relative to sons (Hypothesis 1b).

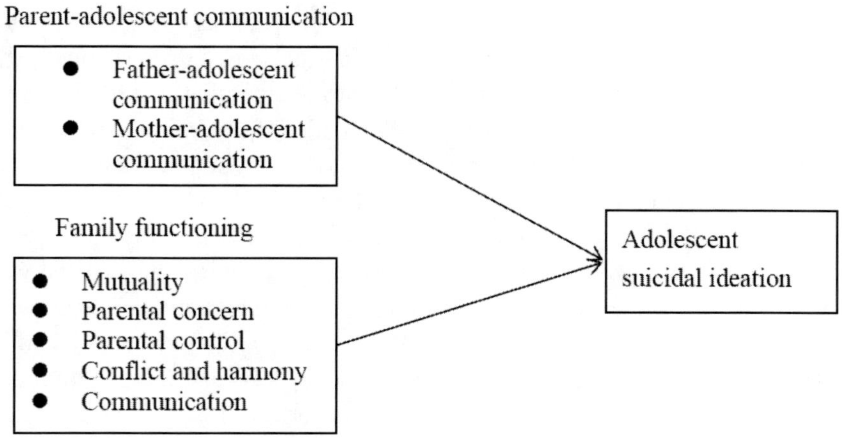

Figure 1. Conceptual framework on the relationship between parent-adolescent communication and family functioning and adolescent suicidal ideation.

The second question is: what is the relationship between perceived family functioning and adolescent suicidal ideation? Based on the prediction of family systems theory that individuals are affected by the family system as a whole (34) and previous research findings (13,36), it was hypothesized that perceived family functioning would have a negative relationship with adolescent suicidal ideation (Hypothesis 2).

The third research question is: are different dimensions of family functioning (i.e. mutuality, communication, conflict and harmony, parental control, parental concern) differentially related to adolescent suicidal ideation? Based on Western theories of family functioning (e.g. Beaver's and Olson's models) derived from family systems theory, communication is a central family process. As such, it was expected that relative to other aspects of family functioning, communication would have the greatest effect on adolescent suicidal ideation (Hypothesis 3a). On the other hand, as Chinese families emphasize the importance of maintaining harmony, avoiding conflict, promoting family cohesion and mutual support, it was alternatively postulated that "conflict and harmony" would be the most important predictor, followed by mutuality, communication, parental concern, then parental control (Hypothesis 3b).

The fourth research question is: what is the relative importance of parent-adolescent communication and family functioning in predicting adolescent suicidal ideation? As previous studies yield controversial results, it is theoretically and practically interesting to explore the relative importance of dyadic communication and systemic family functioning in predicting adolescent suicidal ideation.

OUR STUDY

A cross-sectional survey was conducted and convenience sampling was used. School social workers helped to contact the principals of the secondary schools in which they stationed. Among the principals of 68 schools (out of a total of 426 secondary schools in Hong Kong) being contacted, those from 42 schools (including self-financed, subvented and government schools) from Hong Kong Island, Kowloon, and the New Territories agreed to join the study. The response rate was 62%, which is comparable with other similar studies on suicidal ideation and behavior (37,38). By the end of the survey period, a total of 5,557 valid questionnaires had been collected. With reference to the total secondary student population in Hong Kong at the time the study was conducted (328,573 students), the sample size used (2% of the total secondary student population) can be regarded as adequate and the gender and form ratios in the sample were similar to those based on the population. There were slightly more males (53.1%) than females (46.9%) in the sample, which reflects the distribution among the general population. The participants were evenly distributed among different forms (25.8% in Grade 7, 24.7% in Grade 8, 24.4% in Grade 9, 25.1% in Grade 10). The age of the respondents varied from 11 to 18 years, with an overall mean of 13.87 years (SD = 1.47).

Parent consent letters were sent to the parents to explain the purpose of the study and get their consent prior to the survey. During the survey, a school social worker, a teacher or a research assistant was present to give a short briefing on the general aims and the confidentiality of the study. It was clearly stated that participation in the study was voluntary and they could refuse to complete the questionnaires if so desired. Refusal to join the study would carry no subsequent penalty. Consent forms were signed by those participating students.

The research assistants, but not the teachers nor the social workers, were present throughout the whole administration process to answer queries raised by the participants. The administration process took around 40 minutes to complete. Since the questionnaires were anonymous, individual participants could not be identified.

To facilitate follow up work by the school social workers, individual school reports were sent to the workers so that they could identify classes with more students having higher suicidal ideation and hold prevention groups and programs.

INSTRUMENTS

- *Parent-adolescent communication.* Parent-adolescent communication was assessed using the father-adolescent communication scale (FACS) and mother-adolescent communication scale (MACS) developed by Shek et al. (23). Each instrument contains 25 identical items and assesses the quality of parent-adolescent communication with either the father or mother (e.g., "I can voice out my thinking and feeling to my father/mother in our communication"; "Father/mother knows my feeling even when he/she has not asked me"). As the Chinese are not used to express their feelings, there are eight items in the scale to explore this phenomenon descriptively. A higher FACS or MACS score indicates a higher level of quality of parent-adolescent communication. Moreover, Shek et al. (23) reported that the two measures were able to discriminate adolescents with good and bad communication with their parents, thus lending support to the criterion-related validity of the measure. The scale had significant correlation with adolescent psychological well-being (i.e. mastery and life satisfaction). Reliability analyses showed that the FACS and MACS had high reliability in this study (α =.93 and .94, respectively).

- *Family functioning.* Family functioning was assessed using the Chinese Family Assessment Instrument (C-FAI), which is one of the first indigenous instrument designed to measure family functioning in Chinese families (39). For each question, respondents were required to choose an answer from a 5-point Likert scale. There are five subscales: Mutuality (e.g. family members accommodate each other), Communication (e.g. family members enjoy getting together), Conflict and Harmony (e.g. there is much friction among family members), Parental Concern (parents take care of their children) and Parental Control (e.g. parents force children to do things). A higher score in the five subscales indicates a higher level of family functioning. On closer examination of the dimensions of the C-FAI, the Mutuality, Communication, and Parental Concern factors represent dimensions related to cohesiveness and communication in Western literature. The Conflict and Harmony dimension was a distinct dimension of family functioning in Hong Kong Chinese families, reflecting the importance attributed to the "absence of conflict", which was regarded by the Chinese parents and children as an attribute of happy families in Hong Kong (28). The other two dimensions, Parental Concern and Parental Control were related to functioning of parents, which suggested that parents were quite influential in family functioning in the Chinese families. A series of large-sample validation studies were conducted (40,41) which provided strong support for the psychometric properties of the scale. It was found that there was moderate correlation between C-FAI and parent adolescent conflict measured by Conflict Behavior Questionnaire. The scale was demonstrated to have high reliability in this study (α =.93).
- *Suicidal ideation.* Adolescent suicidal ideation was assessed using the Suicidal Ideation Sub-Scale (C-SIS) of the Suicidal Risk Scale for Hong Kong students developed by Tse (42). The instrument is used as a screening tool to identify high-risk students so that effective intervention can be implemented. In addition, it is used for assessment of suicidal risk during the intervention phase and evaluation of the effectiveness of intervention and treatment programs. The C-SIS contains 13 items (e.g., "I really want to put an end to all this so that I don't have to continue to bear the pain"; "Some problems can only be solved by death"). Chinese tended to use escape and avoidance when facing problems, and might regard death as the only way out when the problem could not be solved (43). For each item, respondents were required to choose an answer from a 4-point Likert scale ranging from "*strongly agree*" to "*strongly disagree*". A higher score indicates a higher level of suicidal ideation. Previous findings based on a validation study (42) showed that the C-SIS has high internal consistency (α = .92), split-half consistency (α = .88) and test-retest reliability (r = .72). In the study of construct validity by Tse and Bagley (42), C-SIS displayed significant relationships with other related measures such as Suicide Behavior Questionnaire (44) and the CES-D (45). Moreover, the C-SIS scores were able to discriminate suicidal and non-suicidal students, with a significant t-value of -

23.26 ($p < .001$). Reliability analyses showed that the scale had high reliability in this study ($\alpha = .93$).

- *Parents' demographics*. As previous studies demonstrated that parents' education level and family income were significant predictors of adolescent suicidal ideation (46,47) they were incorporated as covariates in hierarchical regression analyses of the current study.

OUR FINDINGS

The mean total scores for the Father-adolescent Communication Scale, Mother-adolescent Communication Scale, Chinese Family Assessment Instrument, and Suicidal Ideation Sub-Scale (C-SIS) were 60.45 (SD = 13.49), 69.27 (SD = 13.92), 118.72 (SD = 24.34), and 22.54 (SD = 8.64), respectively. Although there was no clinical cut-off score for C-SIS, about 9.3% of the sample had a raw score of 35 or above, which was a relatively high score as defined by Tse's study (42). Hence, a score of 35 or above indicates high levels of suicidal ideation in this study. Pearson correlation analyses showed that there was significant correlation among father-adolescent communication, mother-adolescent communication, family functioning, male and female adolescent suicidal ideation (Table 1).

Research Question 1: Pearson correlation analyses supported Hypothesis 1 that perceived parent-adolescent communication would have a negative relationship with adolescent suicidal ideation. The relationship between mother-adolescent communication and suicidal ideation was higher than father-adolescent communication and suicidal ideation in the male sample (t = 4.76, p <.001) and the female sample (t = 4.34, p <.001) (Table 1), thus providing some support for Hypothesis 1a. Further analysis showed that the relationship between father-adolescent communication and suicidal ideation in the male respondents was weaker than that in the female respondents (t = 2.99, p < .01), which gives support to Hypothesis 1b. Moreover, hierarchical regression analyses were performed. Demographic variables (including fathers' and mothers' education, monthly family income), parent-adolescent communication (including father-adolescent communication, mother-adolescent communication), family functioning (including mutuality, communication, conflict and harmony, parental concern, parental control) were entered in hierarchical blocks.

Table 1. Correlations among father-adolescent communication, mother-adolescent communication, family functioning and adolescent suicidal ideation split by gender

	Father-adolescent communication	Mother-adolescent communication	Family functioning	Adolescent suicidal ideation
Father-adolescent communication	--	.37***	.65***	-.39***
Mother-adolescent communication	.41***	--	.67***	-.43***
Family functioning	.66***	.66***	--	-.48***
Adolescent suicidal ideation	-.33***	-.42***	-.43***	--

*p < .05, **p <.01, ***p <.001, correlation coefficients for females above diagonal and males below diagonal.

It was found that the fathers' education was a significant predictor of adolescent suicidal ideation, although the related effect size was small. It was also shown that father-adolescent communication (β = -.13, p < .001) and mother- adolescent communication predicted adolescent suicidal ideation (β = -.23, p < .001), explaining 22% of the variance in the total sample when the demographic characteristics were controlled (Table 2). However, some gender and parental differences in the relationship between parent-adolescent communication and suicidal ideation were identified.

First, father-adolescent communication exerted a stronger effect on daughters (β = -.16) than sons (β = -.10), z = 3.71, p < .001. Second, parental differences in the linkage between the two domains were found. In the male respondents, mother-son communication had a stronger linkage with suicidal ideation than did father-son communication (t = 8.54, p <.001).

Among the female respondents, mother-daughter communication similarly had a stronger linkage with suicidal ideation than did father-daughter communication (t = 4.69, p < .01). These findings provide support for Hypothesis 1b.

Table 2. Hierarchical multiple regression analysis for the prediction of adolescent suicidal ideation in the total sample

	Step 1 (β)	Step 2 (β)	Step 3 (β)
Fathers' education[a]	-.06**	-.03	-.03
Mothers' education	.002	.03	.02
Family income	-.03	-.002	.01
Father-adolescent communication		-.23***	-.13***
Mother-adolescent communication			
Mutuality		-.35***	-.23***
Communication			
Conflict & harmony			-.10**
Parental concern			-.04
Parental control			-.16***
			-.14***
			-.08***
F	8.20	205.45	144.33
R^2	.01	.23	.28
Change in R^2		.22	.05

Note: β = Standardized regression coefficient

[a]**Fathers' education** (1= Primary education or below, 2= Secondary education, 3= Tertiary education or above).

**p < .01, ***p < .001.

Research Question 2: Pearson correlation analyses with Bonferroni-corrected alpha levels were performed. There was also support for Hypothesis 2 that perceived family functioning would be negatively related to adolescent suicidal ideation. Specifically, adolescent suicidal ideation was negatively related to mutuality, communication, conflict and harmony, parental concern and parental control (r = -.39, -.36, -.44, -.39, -.39, p<.0083) (Table 3).

Table 3. Correlation coefficients on the relationships between measures of family functioning and adolescent suicidal ideation

Suicidal ideation	Mutuality	Communi-cation	Conflict & harmony	Parental concern	Parental control	Total
Male	-.36*	-.33*	-.44*	-.40*	-.38*	-.43*
Female	-.43*	-.39*	-.44*	-.39*	-.41*	-.48*
Total	-.39*	-.36*	-.44*	-.39*	-.39*	-.46*

*p<.0083 (Bonferroni –corrected alpha level).
Pconcern= parental concern Pcontrol= parental control.
*p<.05 **p<.01 ***p<.001.

Research Question 3: Analyses showed that the level of multicollinearity within different family predictors of adolescent suicidal ideation is acceptable in the current study, with all variation inflation factors (VIFs) below 10 (48). Among the five dimensions of family functioning, hierarchical regression analysis showed that mutuality, "conflict and harmony", parental concern and parental control were significant predictors of adolescent suicidal ideation (Table 2).

Contrary to the prediction of Western family theories, communication was not a significant predictor (i.e. no support for Hypothesis 3a). Further analyses showed that there were no significant differences among the betas of different dimensions of family functioning and suicidal ideation (Table 4). Hence, mutuality, "conflict and harmony", parental concern, parental control had similar importance in predicting suicidal ideation (i.e. no support for Hypothesis 3b). In addition, it was shown that family functioning predicted an additional 5% of the variance in the total sample.

Research Question 4: A comparison of the regression coefficients of the dyadic and systemic variables showed that both family functioning (t = 6.06 , p<.001) and mother-adolescent communication (t = 7.96 . p<.001) were stronger predictors of suicidal ideation than was father-adolescent communication, while there were no significant differences between mother-adolescent communication and family functioning in predicting suicidal ideation (Table 5). Hence, both dyadic (at least for mother-adolescent communication) and systemic factors have similar importance in predicting adolescent suicidal ideation.

Table 4. Comparison of the strength of relationships (beta coefficients) between different dimensions of family functioning and suicidal ideation

	Mutuality & SI	Conflict, Harmony & SI	P concern & SI	P control & SI
Mutuality & SI	-			
Conflict, Harmony & SI	-.10 vs. -.16, t=1.70	-		
P concern & SI	-.10 vs, -.14, t=0.92	-.16 vs. -.14, t=0.41	-	
P control & SI	-.10 vs, -.08, t=0.28	-.16 vs. -.08, t=1.79	-	-

Note: SI = suicidal ideation; Pconcern = parental concern; Pcontrol= parental control.

Table 5. Comparison of the strength of association (beta coefficients) between dyadic and systemic family processes and adolescent suicidal ideation

	Family functioning & suicidal ideation	Father-adolescent communication & suicidal ideation	Mother-adolescent communication & suicidal ideation
Family functioning & suicidal ideation	-		
Father-adolescent communication & suicidal ideation	-.22 vs. -.13 t=6.06***	-	
Mother-adolescent communication & suicidal ideation	-.22 vs. -.23 t=1.36	-.13 vs. -.23 t=7.96***	-

*** $p<.001$.

DISCUSSION

In response to the limitations in the related literature, there are several unique features of the present study. First, Chinese adolescents were recruited in this study. Second, a large sample based on Grade 7 to Grade 10 students was employed. Third, locally developed and validated measures of parent-adolescent communication, family functioning and suicidal ideation were used. Fourth, relationship between father-son, father-daughter, mother-son and mother-daughter communications and adolescent suicidal ideation was explored, while the relative impact of father-adolescent communication and mother-adolescent communication on adolescent suicidal ideation was examined. Fifth, the relative importance of different dimensions of family functioning on adolescent suicidal ideation was studied. Finally, the relative importance of dyadic and systemic process in predicting adolescent suicidal ideation was examined. Practically, it has implications on the different roles played by fathers and mothers in preventing adolescent suicidal ideation and how adolescents with suicidal ideation should be treated (e.g. family therapy or individual counseling).

Results indicated that fathers' education impacted adolescent suicidal ideation, which corroborates previous findings (46). Fathers with better education were found to be more confident in parenting, more respectful of their children, and more warm and involved in child rearing. Since suicidal adolescents perceived their parents to be significantly more critical and less caring, educated parents who were more caring would inevitably have a better relationship with their children, which could have a positive impact on adolescents' psychological well-being and lower their suicidal ideation.

Both correlation and regression analysis showed that a higher level of parent-adolescent communication was significantly related to a lower level of adolescent suicidal ideation, thus giving support for Hypothesis 1. This observation is in line with research findings that there were less frequent and less satisfying parent-adolescent communications among suicidal adolescents (49). Moreover, this observation is consistent with the prediction of family systems theory (34) that parent-child interaction is a determinant of a child's psychological well-being. When the male and female respondents were compared, father-adolescent communication appeared to have a stronger impact on girls than boys, thus supporting Hypothesis 1a. This finding is consistent with the research findings in the United States. Herrara, Dahlblom, Dahlgren, and Kullgren (50) reported that the absence of the father in the family contributed strongly to daughters' suicidal behavior. Both United States and Hong

Kong studies showed that adolescent girls were more susceptible to the influence of family than were adolescent boys (e.g. 26, 27). Due to difference in communication styles with the boys, girls may like to express themselves more and share their problems with the fathers, who may stimulate them to think out solutions with different perspectives. On the contrary, boys are more reserved and are less likely to share things and problems with others, especially the same sex fathers. Therefore, negative parent-adolescent communication would exert a stronger impact for girls than for boys. This finding suggests that gender of children should be taken into account in understanding the impact of fathers on child developmental outcomes.

For both male and female respondents, mother-adolescent communication correlated more highly with suicidal ideation than father-adolescent communication which gives partial support to Hypothesis 1b. This is in line with previous studies that suicide attempters reported significantly less mutuality and communication with their mothers than their fathers (e.g. 51). Traditionally, fathers performed the breadwinner role, while mothers played the socialization and care-giving roles in Chinese society. These traditional gender role differences contribute to mothers' spending more time with the children, while fathers spending more time at work. Furthermore, Chinese women are more encouraged to express their thinking and emotions, and are better listeners than men. Hence, adolescents like to communicate with their mothers more than their fathers. These cultural conditions may explain why mother-adolescent communication was regarded as more important for the adolescents than father-adolescent communication (23). Theoretically speaking, the findings underscore the complexity of the relationship between parent-adolescent communication and adolescent suicidal ideation, and highlight that gender and parental differences should be taken into account. Furthermore, it is possible that parents may have different impacts on adolescents, depending on the nature of outcome indicators under focus.

Results also showed that perceived healthy family functioning is negatively related to adolescent suicidal ideation supporting Hypothesis 2. This is consistent with the prediction of the family systems theory that family functioning is closely linked to a child's psychological well being (34). It also corroborates previous finding that poorer family functioning was significantly correlated with higher suicidal ideation (52). Among the five dimensions of family functioning, mutuality is one of the significant predictors of adolescent suicidal ideation. As Chinese families emphasize family cohesion, mutual trust and support among the family members, adolescents living in families lacking mutuality may feel lonely and frustrated, thus increasing their suicidal ideation.

With reference to Hypothesis 3a, it is interesting to note that communication in the whole family was not a significant predictor for adolescent suicidal ideation. This is not consistent with the prediction of Western family models (e.g. 36,53) and previous studies (23) that emphasize the role of communication within the family. This puzzle may be due to the methodological characteristic of the study. Some of the items in the instrument asked the respondents whether their family members usually arranged family activities, enjoyed getting together and talking to one another. As the adolescents at their developmental stage usually enjoyed getting together and having activities with their peers rather than family members, family activities might not be regarded as important. This explains why communication in the family is not an important predictor of adolescent suicidal ideation.

The finding that "conflict and harmony" significantly predicts adolescent suicidal ideation is in line with previous findings (10,54). Traditionally, Chinese people emphasized avoidance of interpersonal conflict and cultivation of interpersonal harmony, as revealed in the Chinese cultural sayings, "If a family lives in harmony, everything will prosper. A family will wither if there are many quarrels". Confucianism emphasized social and family harmony (55,56). Chinese families were generally thought to be highly cohesive, partially due to a strong cultural emphasis on harmony and mutual obligations, with low value placed on overt expressions of affection and disapproval. Obedience and respect for the authority were valued and conflicts in the families were suppressed (57). Hence, overt conflict in the family, particularly parent-adolescent conflict, would cause disturbance and stress to the adolescents, affecting their psychological well-being (e.g. sense of hope, satisfaction with life), thus increasing their suicidal ideation (27). However, the findings did not provide support for Hypothesis 3b.

Results of the study showed that parental concern was also a strong predictor of adolescent suicidal ideation. As adolescents experienced a period of storm and turmoil, they still needed a lot of emotional support from their parents. Hence, parental concern was important and positively related to adolescents' psychological adjustment and well-being (58), which would also affect their suicidal ideation. Furthermore, parental control was another important predictor of adolescent suicidal ideation. It is understandable that adolescents, who strive for freedom and independence, would resist parental control. Previous studies showed that the adolescent suicide attempters perceived their parents to be less affectionate and more controlling with them than their siblings (e.g. 59). A Hong Kong study also found that parental psychological control was negatively related to adolescent psychological well-being (60). Hence, parental control would affect adolescents' psychological well-being, which contributed to suicidal ideation.

When comparing dyadic and systemic impacts with reference to research question 4, it was found that both mechanisms have similar predictive power on adolescent suicidal ideation. Although general family functioning affects adolescents, parent-adolescent communication has similar impacts. In Chinese families, parent-child communication and relationship are emphasized more than sibling or other familial relationship. Positive encouragement, support and concern from parents are more treasured by the children, though family support, cohesion and harmony also play an important role in a child's development. Hence, it can be understood that the relative importance of dyadic and systemic factors in predicting adolescent suicidal ideation is similar.

IMPLICATIONS

As this study underscores the important role of the following features: parent-adolescent communication (particularly mother-adolescent communication), family functioning (particularly mutuality, parental concern, parental control, conflict and harmony) in adolescent suicidal ideation; these features should be considered as the key building blocks in theoretical models, particularly family models, for adolescent suicidal ideation. The present findings are important because there are few theoretical models on the family determinants of adolescent behavior in the Chinese context (35). As theoretical models on the family determinants of adolescent suicidal ideation are almost non-existent in the Chinese cultural contexts, the present findings are pioneering contribution to the literature.

As the present findings suggest that it is important to enhance parent-adolescent communication, several practice possibilities for preventing adolescent suicidal ideation can be considered in this context. First, parallel groups for both the parents and adolescents enhancing the communication skills in parents and adolescents (61) could be considered. This facilitates reciprocal changes both in the parents and the adolescents. Second, manual-based parenting program, such as the Systematic Training for Effective Parenting Program designed by Dinkmeyer and McKay, based on Adlerian psychology, could be introduced to improve parent-adolescent relationship (62). Manual-based training program conducted by professionals is suitable for Chinese parents because they tend to listen to authoritative figures and adhere to systematic training. This can facilitate them to learn new concepts and skills, e.g. assertive communication.

However, it should be noted that communication and emotional expressiveness were not emphasized in traditional Chinese families (23). Parents and adolescents, especially the fathers and the sons, might feel uneasy or embarrassed to express emotional issues. Direct and open expression of feelings, particularly negative feelings, may be interpreted as blaming. Moreover, parents like to use double-bind messages rather than clear and specific statements, and are accustomed to use name-calling and put-down words rather than express their worries and concern.

Based on the above discussion and the literature on Chinese family intervention, the following content for Chinese parent communication groups is suggested. Parents are guided to: (a) respect and trust the adolescents, (b) provide more opportunity as well as a free and relaxing environment for communication, (c) take initiatives to express their concern to the adolescents, (d) be willing to listen to what the adolescents say; look at things from the adolescents' perspectives, (e) reflect on the adolescents' thinking and feeling, (f) guide the adolescents to think out different solutions, evaluate their pros and cons, and let them make decisions, (g) encourage the adolescents to express their thinking and feelings openly, and to raise problems for discussion. The parents should also be guided to avoid ordering, ridiculing, criticizing, provoking, indoctrinating, nagging the adolescents, dominating the discussion and using double-bind messages. In turn, the Chinese adolescents should also be taught to respect and trust their parents, take initiative to communicate with their parents, express their feeling and thinking, look at things from the parents' perspectives, and try to understand the parents' thinking and feeling.

The results also indicated that family functioning, particularly parental concern, parental control, conflict and harmony and mutuality, were significantly related to adolescent suicidal ideation. Thus, it is important to enhance parental concern, harmony and mutuality, while minimizing parental control and conflict within the family. The Positive Parenting Program for parents, which was effective in promoting harmonious family relationships in Chinese families in Hong Kong, could be organized to strengthen family functioning (63). Nevertheless, care should be taken that excessive parental concern is not mistaken by adolescents for control, so parents should be guided to give an appropriate level of concern to their teenagers. As many mothers get a large part of their life satisfaction from taking care of and controlling their children, they may be quite fearful of losing control over them (64). Hence, it is important for family practitioners to appreciate parents' efforts to take care of their children, but also help them to realize the possible negative impacts of excessive control.

From a systemic perspective, family mutuality and cohesion can be enhanced by guiding the family members to love, care, concern, trust, support and understand one another. They should also be taught to tolerate, forbear, accommodate and be considerate to one another. In addition, family harmony can be achieved by teaching the family members ways to resolve family conflicts and facilitating the couples to enrich their marital relationship. The parents should also be guided to increase parental concern and decrease parental control by understanding adolescents' perception of concern and control.

LIMITATIONS

It is noteworthy that there are several limitations to our study. First, the weaknesses of convenience sampling should be noted. In particular, generalization of the present findings to the secondary school population should proceed with caution. Second, as self-administered questionnaires were used, the information collected was based on the adolescent informants only. If resource permits, the use of multiple informants that know the adolescents would give a clearer picture of the problem area.

Third, the present research predominately used quantitative methodology. In addition, a qualitative study can be conducted to better understand the texture of the relationship between the parents and the adolescents in contributing to adolescent suicidal ideation.

Fourth, only two family correlates (perceived parent-adolescent communication and family functioning) were selected, based on a review of empirical findings and the theoretical framework. Other personal factors (e.g. self-esteem), familial factors (e.g. parenting style, family rules), school factors (such as school performance, relationship with schoolmates) and societal factors (e.g. mass media, social integration) can also be included in future studies of adolescent suicidal ideation.

Fifth, the use of a cross-sectional design means that it is not possible to claim a causal relationship between the antecedents and adolescent suicidal ideation. Hence, a longitudinal research design can be used in future studies.

Despite these limitations, the present study can be regarded as a stimulating and interesting addition to the literature which has enriched our understanding of the relationship between family processes (perceived parent-adolescent communication and family functioning) and Chinese adolescent suicidal ideation.

REFERENCES

[1] Lo PC. Confucian views on suicide. Hong Kong: Centre for Applied Ethics, Hong Kong Baptist University, 1997.

[2] Shek DTL, Lee BM, Chow JTW. Trends in adolescent suicide in Hong Kong for the period of 1980 to 2003. ScientificWorldJournal 2005;5:702-23.

[3] Lam TH, Stewart SM, Yip SF, Leung M, Ho LM, Ho SY, Lee WH. Suicidality and cultural values among Hong Kong adolescents. Soc Sci Med 2004;58: 487-98.

[4] Wong JPS, Stewart SM, Ho SY, Rao U, Lam TH. Exposure to suicide and suicidal behaviors among Hong Kong adolescents. Soc Sci Med 2005;61:591-9.

[5] Lee TY, Wong P, Chow WY, McBride-Chang C. Predictors of suicide ideation and depression in Hong Kong adolescents: Perceptions of academic and family climates. Suicide Life Threat Behav 2006;36:82-97.

[6] Eaton D, Kann L, Kinchen S, Ross J, Hawkins J, Harris W. Youth risk behavior surveillance, United States, 2005. MMWR 2006;55:1-108.

[7] Reinherz HZ, Tanner JL, Berger SR, Beardslee WR, Fitzmaurice GM. Adoelscent suicidal ideation as predictive of psychopathology, suicidal behavior and compromised functioning at age 30. Am J Psychiatry 2006;163(7):1226-32.

[8] Witte TK, Fitzpatrick KK, Joiner TE, Schmidt NB. Variability in suicidal ideation: A better predictor of suicide attempts than intensity or duration of ideation? J Affect Disord 2005;88:131-6.

[9] Lai KW, McBride-Chang C. Suicidal ideation, parenting style, and family climate among Hong Kong adolescents. Int J Psychol 2001;36(2):81-7.

[10] Wong IN, De Man AF, Leung PWL. Perceived parental child rearing and suicidal ideation in Chinese adolescents. Soc Behav Pers 2002;30:19-24.

[11] Coleman H. The relationships between suicidal ideation and three aspects of the self in 18- and 19-year-old college students. ProQuest Information Learning 2008.

[12] Esposito CL, Clum GA. The relative contribution of diagnostic and psychosocial factors in the prediction of adolescent suicidal ideation. J Clin Child Adolesc Psychol 2003;32:386.

[13] Spirito A, Valeri S, Boergers J, Donaldson D. Predictors of continued suicidal behavior in adolescents following a suicide attempt. J Clin Child Adolesc Psychol 2003;32: 284.

[14] Stewart SM, Felice E, Claassen C, Kennard BD, Lee PWH, Emslie GJ. Adolescent suicide attempters in Hong Kong and the United States. Soc Sci Med 2006;63(2):296-306.

[15] Shek DTL. Chinese adolescents and their parents' views on a happy family: Implications for family therapy. Fam Ther 2001;28:73-104.

[16] Mitchell MG, Rosenthal DM. Suicidal adolescents: Family dynamics and the effects of lethality and hopelessness. J Youth Adolesc 1992;21:23-33.

[17] Ponnet K, Vermeiren R, Jespers I, Mussche B, Ruchkin V, Schwab-Stone M, Deboutte D. Suicidal behaviour in adolescents: Associations with parental marital status and perceived parent-adolescent relationship. J Affect Disord 2005;89:107-13.

[18] Shek DTL, Chan LK. Perceptions of a happy family amongst Chinese adolescents and their parents. J Youth Stud 1998;1:178-89.

[19] Ho DYF. Filial piety and its psychological consequences. In: Bond MH, ed. The handbook of Chinese psychology. Hong Kong: Oxford University Press, 1996;155-65.

[20] Shek DTL, Lai MF. Conceptions of an ideal family in Confucian thoughts: Implications for individual and family counseling. Asian J Couns 2000;7:85-104.

[21] Ho DYF. Chinese patterns of socialization: A critical review. In: Bond MH, ed. The psychology of the Chinese People. Oxford: Oxford University Press, 1986.

[22] Landman-Peeters KMC, Hartman CA, van de Pompe G, den Boer JA, Minderaa RB, Ormel J. Gender differences in the relation between social support, problem in parent-offspring communication, and depression and anxiety. Soc Sci Med 2005;60:2549-255.

[23] Shek DTL, Lee TY, Lee BM, Chow J. Perceived parental control and psychological well-being in Chinese adolescents in Hong Kong. Int J Adolesc Med Health 2006;18:535-45.

[24] Adams DM, Overholser JC, Lehnert KL. Perceived family functioning and adolescent suicidal behavior. J Am Acad Child Adolesc Psychiatry 1994;33:4-11.

[25] King CA, Hill EM, Naylor MT, Shain EB. Alcohol consumption in relation to other predictors of suicidality among adolescent inpatient girls. J Am Acad Child Adolesc Psychiatry 1993;32:82-8.

[26] Houck CD, Rodrigue JR, Lobato D. Parent-adolescent communication and psychological symptoms among adolescents with chronically ill parents. J Pediatr Psychol 2007;32:596-604.

[27] Shek DTL. A longitudinal study of the relations of family functioning to adolescent psychological well-being. J Youth Stud 1998;1:195-209.

[28] Rosnati R, Lafrate R, Scabini E. Parent-adolescent communication in foster, inter-country adoptive, and biological Italian families: Gender and generational differences. Int J Psychol 2007;42:36-45.

[29] Shek DTL. Parenting characteristics and adolescent psychological well-being: A longitudinal study in a Chinese context. Genet Soc Gen Psychol Monogr 1999;125:27-44.

[30] Shek DTL. Adolescent developmental issues in Hong Kong: Relevance to positive youth development programs in Hong Kong. In: Shek DTL, Ma HK, Merrick J, eds. Positive youth development: Development of a pioneering program in a Chinese context. London: Freund, 2007:9-23.
[31] Tulloch AL, Blizzard L, Pinkus Z. Adolescent–parent communication in self-harm. J Adolesc Health 1997;21(4):267-75.
[32] Brage D, Meredith W. A causal model of adolescent depression. J Psychol Interdiscip Appl 1994;128(4):455-68.
[33] McDermut W, Miller IW, Solomon D, Ryan CE, Keitner GI. Family functioning and suicidality in depressed adults. Compr Psychiatry 2001;42(2):96-104.
[34] Bowen M. Family therapy in clinical practice. New York: Jason Aronson, 1978.
[35] Shek DTL. Chinese family research: Puzzles, progress, paradigms, and policy implications. J Fam Issues 2006;27:275-84.
[36] Olson DH, Russell CS, Sprenkle DH. Circumplex Model: systemic assessment and treatment of families. New York: Harworth Press, 1989.
[37] Cheung YB, Law CK, Chan B, Liu KY, Yip SF. Suicidal ideation and suicidal attempts in a population-based study of Chinese people: Risk attributable to hopelessness, depression, and social factors. J Affect Disord 2006;90:193-9.
[38] Lynch F, Mills C, Daly I, Fitzpatick C. Challenging times: Prevalence of psychiatric disorders and suicidal behavior in Irish adolescents. J Adolesc 2006;29:555-73.
[39] Shek DTL. Assessment of family functioning in Chinese adolescents. In: Singh NN, ed. International perspectives on child and adolescent mental health. Amsterdam: Elsevier, 2000.
[40] Siu MH, Shek DTL. Psychometric properties of the Chinese Family Assessment Instrument in Chinese adolescent in Hong Kong. Adolesc 2005;40: 817-830.
[41] Shek DTL. Assessment of family functioning in Chinese adolescents: The Chinese version of the Family Assessment Device. Res Soc Work Pract 2002;12:502-24.
[42] Tse WL, Bagley C. Suicidal behavior, bereavement and death education in Chinese adolescents. Burlington, VT: Ashgate, 2002.
[43] Hwang KK. The patterns of coping strategies in a Chinese society. Acta Psychol (Amst) Taiwan 1977;9:61-73.
[44] Linehan MM. Suicidal behaviors questionnaire. Seattle, WA: University Washington, 1981.
[45] Radloff LS. The CES-D scale: A self-report depression scale for research in the general population. Appl Psychol Meas 1977;1:385-401.
[46] Zeng Q. An exploratory study of child development and parenting: A Chinese perspective. ProQuest Information Learning, 1999.
[47] Brent D, Greenhill L, Compton S, Emslie G, Wells K, Walkup T. The treatment of adolescent suicide attempters study (TASA): Predictors of suicidal events in an open treatment trial. J Am Acad Child Adolesc Psychiatry 2009;48(10):987-96.
[48] Myers RH. Classical and modern regression with applications. The Duxbury advanced series in statistics and decision sciences. Boston, MA: PWS-Kent, 1990.
[49] Everall RD, Bostik KE, Paulson BL. Being in the safety zone: Emotional experiences of suicidal adolescents and emerging adults. J Adolesc Res 2006;21:370-92.
[50] Herrara A, Dahlblom K, Dahlgren L, Kullgren J. Pathways to suicidal behavior among adolescent girls in Nicaragua. Soc Sci Med 2006;62:805-14.
[51] Zayas LH, Bright CL, Alvarez-Sanchex T, Cabassa LJ. Acculturation, familism and mother-daughter relations among suicidal and non-suicidal adolescent Latinas. J Prim Prev 2009;30:351-69.
[52] Wagner BM. Family risk factors for child and adolescent suicidal behavior. Psychol Bull 1997;121(2):246-98.
[53] Beavers WR, Hampson RB, Hulgus YF. Manual: Beavers systems model of family assessment. Dallas, TX: Southwest Family Institute, 1990.
[54] Fotti A, Katz Y, Afifi O, Cox J. The associations between peer and parental relationships and suicidal behaviors in early adolescents. Can J Psychiatry 2006;51:698-703.
[55] Ho DYF. Traditional patterns of socialization in Chinese society. Acta Psychol (Amst) Taiwan 1981;23:81-95.

[56] Hsu J. The Chinese family: Relations, problems and therapy. In: Tseng W, Wu DYH, eds. Chinese culture and mental health. Orlando, FL: Academic Press, 1985.

[57] Liang SM. The essential features of Chinese culture. Hong Kong: Chi-Cheng T'u-Shu Kung Shu, 1974.

[58] Shek DTL. Psychological well-being, school adjustment, and problem behavior among Chinese adolescent boys from poor families: Does family functioning matter? In: Way N, Chu JY, eds. Adolescent boys: Exploring diverse cultures of boyhood. New York: New York University Press, 2004.

[59] Silverman MAC. Differential sibling treatment within the family and adolescent suicide attempters. Sci Eng 2004;64(10-B):5234.

[60] Shek DTL, Ma HK, Merrick J. Positive youth development: Development of a pioneering program in a Chinese context. London: Freund, 2007.

[61] Chan KL, Yeung KC, Chu CK, Tsang KY, Leung YK. An evaluative study on the effectiveness of a parent-child parallel group model. Res Soc Work Pract 2002;12: 546-57.

[62] Kwok LYC. Systematic training of effective parenting: Its applicability for Chinese parents of primary school children in Hong Kong. Hong Kong J Soc Work 1994;28: 22-30.

[63] Leung C, Sanders MR, Leung S, Mak R, Lau J. An outcome evaluation of the implementation of the triple P-Positive Parenting Program in Hong Kong. Fam Process 2003;42:531-44.

[64] Ma LC. Parenting distress and parental investment of Hong Kong Chinese parents with a child having an emotional or behavioral problem: A qualitative study. Child Fam Soc Work 2002;7:99-106.

In: Adolescence and Behavior Issues in a Chinese Context
Editors: DTL Shek, RCF Sun and Joav Merrick
ISBN: 978-1-62618-614-9

Chapter 12

COGNITIVE, EMOTIVE AND COGNITIVE-BEHAVIORAL CORRELATES OF SUICIDAL IDEATION AMONG CHINESE ADOLESCENTS IN HONG KONG

Sylvia Y.C.L. Kwok[1] and Daniel T.L. Shek[2-6] *

[1]Department of Applied Social Studies,
The City University of Hong Kong, Hong Kong, PRC
[2]Department of Applied Social Sciences,
The Hong Kong Polytechnic University, Hong Kong, PRC
[3]Public Policy Research Institute,
The Hong Kong Polytechnic University, Hong Kong, PRC
[4]Department of Social Work, East China Normal University,
Shanghai, PRC
[5]Kiang Wu Nursing College of Macau, Macau, PRC
[6]Division of Adolescent Medicine, Department of Pediatrics,
Kentucky Children's Hospital,
University of Kentucky College of Medicine, Lexington, KY, US

ABSTRACT

Utilizing Daniel Goleman's theory of emotional competence, Beck's cognitive theory and Rudd's cognitive-behavioral theory of suicidality, the relationships between hopelessness (cognitive component), social problem solving (cognitive-behavioral component) and emotional competence (emotive component) and adolescent suicidal ideation were examined. Based on the responses of 5,557 Secondary 1 to Secondary 4 students from 42 secondary schools in Hong Kong, results showed that suicidal ideation was positively related to adolescent hopelessness but negatively related to emotional competence and social problem solving. While standard regression analyses showed that all the above variables were significant predictors of suicidal ideation, hierarchical

* Correspondence: Professor Daniel T.L. Shek, PhD, FHKPS, BBS, JP, Chair Professor of Applied Social Sciences, Faculty of Health and Social Sciences, Department of Applied Social Sciences, The Hong Kong Polytechnic University, Room HJ407, Core H, Hunghom, Hong Kong. E-mail: daniel.shek@polyu.edu.hk.

regression analyses showed that hopelessness was the most important predictor of suicidal ideation, followed by social problem solving and emotional competence. Further regression analyses found that all the four subscales of emotional competence, i.e. empathy, social skills, self management of emotions, and utilization of emotions were important predictors of male adolescent suicidal ideation. However, social skill was not a significant predictor of female adolescent suicidal ideation. Standard regression analysis also revealed that all the three subscales of social problem solving, i.e. negative problem orientation, rational problem solving, impulsiveness /carelessness style, were important predictors of suicidal ideation.

Theoretical and practice implications of the findings are discussed.

INTRODUCTION

There are different cognitive, emotive and cognitive-behavioral theories explaining suicidal behaviors. Firstly, Aaron Beck's concept of the "cognitive triad" i.e. negative thoughts about oneself, the future, and others, was central to the cognitive theory of suicide (1). Beck's cognitive perspective also states that hopelessness is the most important clinical variable implicated in suicidal behavior. Empirically, a number of studies also found that there was a significant relationship between hopelessness and suicidality (2). In a longitudinal study of Hong Kong Chinese and Caucasian American adolescents (3), hopelessness was found to be the strongest of cognitive variables in concurrent association with suicidal ideation in bivariate and multivariate models (4). However, some studies found that depression was a more powerful predictor of suicidal ideation than was hopelessness (5). Since depression is a chronic illness and requires long term treatment, this study will focus on examining the significance of hopelessness as a cognitive factor in suicidal ideation for its practical value, with reference to Beck's cognitive theory.

According to Daniel Goleman's theory of emotional competence (6), a person with high emotional intelligence has better emotional self-awareness and higher empathy, is more competent in managing own emotions and handling interpersonal relationship, hence will have better psychological well-being.

Empirical studies also stated that there was an emotional element in suicidal ideation. A number of studies have indicated the importance of emotional expression and emotion regulation (7) in working with acutely suicidal individuals. Previous research also suggested that depressed adolescents had difficulty regulating negative affect and had fewer and less effective strategies for emotion regulation (8). Besides, four emotional competencies were found to be important in understanding how well people deal with stress and avoid poor mental health outcomes: perceiving emotions, managing self-relevant emotions, managing others' emotions, and intention to seek help when in emotional need.

However, a study found that at some high-extremes of temperament, emotion regulation had no impact on suicidality (7). In addition, another study revealed that there were gender differences in the relationship between emotion regulation and depressive symptoms (9). Women with high depressive symptoms were found to exhibit greater attention to emotions, more impaired antirumination emotional repair strategies, and greater reports of depressive symptoms than men with high depressive symptoms. A study of Chinese youth found that the girls were significantly higher than boys in terms of effortful control, affability and negative mood, but lower on surgency and aggression (10). Research also showed that females express emotion more than males, due to maternal behavior (11). Since the findings are equivocal and there are differences in emotional expression for the Chinese males and females, the relationship between emotional competence and adolescent suicidal ideation, with reference to gender differences, is worth to be further examined.

D'Zurilla and Maydeu-Olivares made a distinction between two types of problem solving measures: process measures and outcome measures. As a process measure, social problem solving is a cognitive-behavioral construct which includes problem orientation and problem solving proper (12,13). Theoretically, Rudd (14) also suggested a cognitive-behavioral theory of suicidality, elaborating on Beck's modal theory of psychopathology.

According to Rudd, suicidality was associated with the behavioral system, cognitive system, physiological system and affective system, while social problem solving was one of the cognitive-behavioral constructs. Empirically, studies indicated that social problem solving was closely linked with suicidal behavior (15). However, the literature on the relationship between social problem solving and adolescent suicide is not conclusive. On the one hand, there are research findings showing that suicide attempters showed deficits in problem orientation and had difficulty with the generation of alternatives, decision making and solution implementation and verification (16). On the other hand, there are studies showing no significant problem-solving differences between groups of suicidal psychiatric inpatients, non-suicidal psychiatric inpatients, and community high school students (17). In addition, a study found that female adolescents' lower levels of positive thinking, higher scores on negative problem orientation, and self-focused negative cognitions partially mediated gender differences in depressive symptoms (18).

A study with Hong Kong Chinese students showed that girls tended to cope with failure by seeking social support (19). Another study with Hong Kong secondary school students found that boys had significantly higher scores in rational problem solving and impulsiveness/carelessness style than girls (20). As there are differences in the problem solving strategies for the Chinese males and females, the relationship between social problem solving and adolescent suicidal ideation, with reference to gender differences, needs to be further explored.

Theoretically, emotional competence theory, cognitive theory and cognitive-behavioral theory can be used to examine suicidal ideation. Empirically, although Williams and Pollock (21) highlighted emotional regulation, hopelessness and interpersonal problem solving as mediating factors in suicidal behavior, there are controversial results in the studies on the relative importance of hopelessness, social problem solving and emotional competence in predicting suicidal ideation.

Results in a study examining the relationship between social and emotional competence and mental health (22) revealed that all social and emotional competence measures, including social problem solving skill, effective emotional control, and level of emotional awareness, had significant incremental value over stressful events in predicting social and mental health.

A study showed that both problem solving and emotional discharge, as coping strategies, were negatively related with suicidal behavior (23). Although hopelessness and problem solving deficits were highlighted as psychological processes relevant to the understanding of suicidality, a study showed that problem–solving confidence predicted depressive symptoms and hopelessness, but not suicidal ideation in Asian international students (24).

Some other studies found that even after hopelessness was statistically controlled, emotion-oriented coping remained a significant predictor of suicidal ideation in Western people (25). Since the results are equivocal, it is interesting to examine the relative importance of the emotional, cognitive and cognitive-behavioral factors in predicting suicidal ideation. Previous studies stated that there was significant association between exposure to single parenthood and suicidal behavior (26). Research also highlighted that parents' educational level was associated with adolescents' mental health (27). Hence, it is worthwhile to examine whether the same association was found among Chinese adolescents.

However, there are several limitations intrinsic to the previous studies. First, the studies on the relationship amongst different measures of cognitive, emotive and cognitive-behavioral correlates and adolescent suicidal ideation are inconclusive. Second, few studies have included the cognitive, emotive and cognitive-behavioral components in a single study. However, it can be argued that it is both theoretically and empirically important to include all three correlates in a single study and to assess their relative contribution to adolescent suicidal ideation.

Third, the sample size in the existing studies was either too small or limited to a homogenous sub-sample. Fourth, most of the measuring instruments for the studies conducted in Hong Kong were adapted from the West, which may not be able to capture the essence of the Chinese culture. Fifth, there is a predominance of western studies regarding the relationship between the personal or family quality of life measures and adolescent suicidal ideation.

A survey of the PsycINFO in January 2010 with the search term of "suicidal ideation" showed that while there were 5,323 citations, there were only 63 citations when the search terms of "suicidal ideation" and "Chinese" were used. As Chinese people constitute roughly one-fifth of the world's population, my study is an important contribution to fill the gap.

Against the above background, several research questions were addressed in our study:

- What is the relationship between hopelessness, emotional competence and social problem solving and Chinese adolescent suicidal ideation in Hong Kong? Based on the theoretical frameworks of cognitive theory, emotional competence theory and cognitive-behavioral theory, as well as previous research findings, it was hypothesized that a) hopelessness would have a positive relationship with suicidal ideation (Hypothesis 1), b) emotional competence would have a negative relationship with suicidal ideation (Hypothesis 2), and c) social problem solving would have a negative relationship with suicidal ideation (Hypothesis 3).
- What is the relative importance of the above correlates in predicting Chinese adolescent suicidal ideation in Hong Kong? Since previous studies highlighted the significant role of hopelessness in predicting suicidal behavior (4,28), it was hypothesized that hopelessness would be the most important predictor of suicidal ideation. However, as Chinese people may not place too much emphasis on emotional expression when compared with the Western ones, emotion may occupy a relatively less important position (29). Hence, it was hypothesized that emotional competence would be the least important predictor of suicidal ideation (Hypothesis 4).

OUR STUDY

A cross-sectional survey was conducted and secondary schools were approached by convenience sampling with the help of agencies providing school social work service. Of the 68 schools (out of a total of 426 secondary schools in Hong Kong) that were contacted, 42 schools (among these self-financed, subvented and government schools) from Hong Kong Island, Kowloon, and the New Territories agreed to join the study. The response rate was 62%, which is comparable with similar study on suicidal ideation and behavior (22).

By the end of the survey period, a total of 5,557 valid questionnaires had been collected. With reference to the total secondary student population in Hong Kong at the time the study was conducted (328,573 students), the sample size used (2%) can be regarded as adequate. There were slightly more males (53.1%) than females (46.9%) in the sample, which reflects the distribution among the general population.

The participants were evenly distributed among different forms (25.8% in Secondary 1, 24.7% in Secondary 2, 24.4% in Secondary 3, 25.1% in Secondary 4). The age of the respondents varied from 11 to 18 years, with an overall mean of 13.87 years ($SD = 1.47$). A large proportion (81.0%) of the participants reported their fathers to have a full-time job, while 10.0% had part-time job and 9.0% were homemakers or unemployed. A small proportion (23.7%) of the fathers had primary or no education, while 66.4% received secondary education and 9.9% received tertiary education or above. Meanwhile, 42.3% of the mothers had a full-time job, while 15.6% had part-time job and 42.0% were homemakers or unemployed. About one-quarter (26.1%) of the mothers had primary or no education, while 67.4% received secondary education and 6.4% received tertiary education or above. A large proportion (87.7%) of the families of the participants was reported to be intact, and 12.3% reported having non-intact families (i.e. single-parent families due to death of a parent, divorce or separation). About one-third (35.6%) of the participants had a family monthly income lower than HK$10,000 (about US$1,282). A small proportion (13.1%) of the participants' families received Comprehensive Social Security Assistance (CSSA).

School, parental and participant consent were obtained prior to data collection. During the survey, a school social worker, a teacher or a research assistant was present to give a short briefing on the general aims and the confidentiality of the study. They were present throughout the whole administration process to answer queries raised by the participants. Briefing the participants and filling out the questionnaires took around 40 minutes.

Instruments

Hopelessness Subscale of the Chinese Hopelessness Scale (C-HOPE)

The original English scale was devised by Beck, Weissman, Lester, and Trexler (30), and then translated to Chinese and further developed by Shek (31). The subscale has 10 items and the respondents were asked to choose an answer from a 4-point Likert scale ranging from "strongly agree" to "strongly disagree", with a minimum total score of 10 and a maximum total score of 40. A higher score indicates a higher degree of hopelessness. According to Shek and Lee's study (32), the scale possessed adequate construct validity. The scale was demonstrated to be internally consistent in this study ($\alpha = .88$).

Short form of Chinese Emotional Intelligence Scale (C-EIS-R)

Developed by Chan (33), the instrument was adapted from the English 33-item EIS originally developed by Schutte and colleagues (34). The short form of the 12-item C-EIS-R has four empirical subscales to represent four dimensions of emotional intelligence: Self-management of emotions, social skills, empathy and utilization of emotions. Respondents indicate their agreement to each of the 12 statements using a five-point scale ranging from “strongly agree” to “strongly disagree”, with a minimum total score of 12 and a maximum total score of 60. A higher score indicates better emotional competence. The scale was found to be internally consistent in this study ($\alpha = .79$).

Short form of Chinese version of the Social Problem Solving Inventory (C-SPSI-R)

Developed by Siu and Shek (35), the instrument was adapted from the 52-item Social Problem-Solving Inventory Revised (SPSI-R)(11). A validation study was conducted locally with 352 secondary school students (35). The short form of the 25-item C-SPSI-R had a five-factor structure that was largely consistent with the original English SPSI-R. However, the three-factor model of the C-SPSI (35) was used in this study because the subscales had adequate coverage on the social problem solving concept and the internal consistency of the three subscales was good. The three subscales are negative problem orientation (NPO), rational problem solving (RPS), impulsiveness / carelessness style (ICS). For each of the 25 items, the respondents are requested to choose an answer on a 5-point Likert scale ranging from “Not at all true of me” to “Extremely true of me”. In calculating the total score of C-SPSI-R, the items in the subscales of NPO and ICS were reversed, resulting with a minimum total score of 0 and a maximum total score of 100. Half of the test items indicate a constructive orientation toward problem solving, while the other half indicates a dysfunctional or inhibitive orientation.

The items are presented in a random order. A higher score indicates better social competence. There were findings showing that the related measure were valid and reliable (35). Reliability analyses showed that this abridged version of C-SPSI-R was reliable in this study ($\alpha = .83$).

Suicidal Ideation Sub-Scale (C-SIS) of the Suicidal Risk Scale

The scale was locally developed by Tse and Bagley (36). For each of the 13 items, respondents were required to choose an answer from a 4-point Likert scale ranging from “strongly agree” to “strongly disagree” , with a minimum total score of 13 and a maximum total score of 52. A higher score indicates a higher level of suicidal ideation.

A previous validation study (36) showed that the C-SIS has high reliability and validity. Reliability analyses showed that the scale had high reliability in this study ($\alpha = .93$).

Statistical analyses

The means, standard deviations and Cronbach’s alpha (α) were first computed. Then, Pearson correlation analyses between the independent variables of the subscales of emotional competence, subscales of social problem solving, hopelessness, and the dependent variable of suicidal ideation were carried out, using Bonferroni-corrected alpha level to adjust for multiple comparisons. To examine the relative importance within the subscales of emotional competence and social problem solving in predicting suicidal ideation between the two genders, regression analyses were carried out separately for both genders and the total sample. Lastly, to examine the relative importance of emotional competence, social problem solving and hopelessness in predicting suicidal ideation, hierarchical regression analyses were performed. For the first step, socio-demographic variables (including participants' age, fathers' and mothers' jobs, fathers' and mothers' education, parents' marital status, monthly family income, comprehensive social security allowance recipients) were entered as control. For the second step, emotional competence and social problem solving were entered into the equation to determine whether they added significant incremental validity to the prediction model. For the final step, hopelessness was entered into the equation to determine its effects on emotional competence and social problem solving. Linear Mixed Model analysis was also performed to examine whether there was any school or banding effects.

OUR FINDINGS

The mean total scores for the Chinese Hopelessness Scale, Chinese Emotional Intelligence Scale, Social Problem Solving Inventory and Suicidal Ideation Sub-Scale were 20.28 (*SD* = 5.96), 43.95 (*SD* = 6.04), 48,29 (*SD* = 11.51), 22.54 (*SD* = 8.64) respectively (Table 1).

Using Pearson correlation analysis, results showed that there was significant positive correlation between adolescent suicidal ideation and hopelessness ($r = .68$, $p < .001$), hence supporting hypothesis 1. Adolescent suicidal ideation increased when hopelessness increased. Standard regression analysis showed that hopelessness was a significant predictor of adolescent suicidal ideation ($R^2 = .47$).

Table 1. Descriptive statistics of adolescent suicidal ideation, emotional competence, social problem solving, the subscales, and hopelessness in male, female and total sample

	Male		Female		Total		
	M	*SD*	*M*	*SD*	*M*	*SD*	α
Adolescent Suicidal Ideation	22.49	8.63	22.59	8.64	22.54	8.64	.93
Emotional Competence	43.74	6.43	44.18	5.54	43.95	6.04	.79
Self Management of Emotions	11.36	2.20	11.17	2.03	11.27	2.12	.64
Social skills	11.21	2.16	11.81	1.84	11.49	2.04	.64
Empathy	10.63	2.34	10.98	2.01	10.79	2.20	.71
Utilization of Emotions	10.50	2.21	10.20	2.00	10.36	2.12	.64
Social Problem Solving	48.84	11.83	47.68	11.12	48.29	11.51	.83
Negative Problem Orientation	28.63	8.55	28.44	8.26	28.54	8.41	.87
Rational Problem Solving	14.86	5.50	13.56	5.06	14.25	5.33	.84
Impulsiveness / Carelessness Style	5.34	2.02	5.68	1.88	5.50	1.96	.66
Hopelessness	20.66	6.15	19.85	5.73	20.28	5.96	.88

According to Pearson correlation analysis with a Bonferroni-corrected alpha level, there was significant negative correlation between adolescent suicidal ideation and emotional competence ($r = -.19$, $p < .01$). Further analysis showed that there were significant negative correlations between suicidal ideation and three emotional intelligence subscales, self-management of emotions, social skills, utilization of emotions (*r* = -.22, *r* = -.13, *r* = -.17 respectively, $p < .01$) (Table 2), providing partial support for hypothesis 2. However, there was no significant correlation between the empathy subscale and adolescent suicidal ideation. Adolescent suicidal ideation increased when there were lower scores in self-management of emotions, social skills and utilization of emotions.

Since empathy was found to be negatively correlated with suicidal ideation in previous studies (37), this variable will be kept in the subsequent regression analysis. Standard regression analysis showed that emotional competence was a significant predictor of suicidal ideation ($R^2 = .07$). There were no significant differences between the beta coefficients for male and female adolescent suicidal ideation.

Increases in all the subscales of emotional competence, except empathy, were related to a significant decrease in adolescent suicidal ideation. All the four subscales were important predictors of male adolescent suicidal ideation, but only self management of emotions, empathy, and utilization of emotions were important predictors of female adolescent suicidal ideation (see table 3). Pearson correlation analyses with Bonferroni-corrected alpha level were also performed for social problem solving. Results showed that there was a significant negative correlation between adolescent suicidal ideation and social problem solving (*r* = -.37, $p < .0125$). Further analysis revealed that suicidal ideation was significantly related to the three subscales of social problem solving scale, including negative problem orientation, rational problem solving, and impulsiveness/carelessness style (*r* = .30, *r* = -.22, *r* = .23, respectively, $p < .0125$) (see table 4). Hence, hypothesis 3 was supported. Adolescent suicidal ideation increased when there was less rational problem solving, but more negative problem orientation and impulsiveness / carelessness style.

Table 2. Correlations between emotional competence and adolescent suicidal ideation

	Self-management of Emotions	Social Skills	Empathy	Utilization of Emotions	Total
Adolescent Suicidal Ideation	-.22*	-.13*	-.03	-.17*	-.19*

*$p < .01$ (Bonferroni –corrected alpha level).

Table 3. Prediction of adolescent suicidal ideation from emotional competence

Suicidal Ideation			Emotional	competence		
	SME (β)	SS (β)	EM (β)	UE (β)	R^2	*Adj.* R^2
Male	-.18***	-.09***	.10***	-.05*	.05	.05
Female	-.22***	-.04	.11***	-.16***	.09	.09
Total	-.20***	-.07***	.11***	-.10***	.07	.07

Note: β = Standardized regression coefficient SME= self management of emotions SS= social skills EM= empathy UE= utilization of emotions.

*$p < .05$, **$p < .01$, ***$p < .001$.

Table 4. Correlations between social problem solving and adolescent suicidal ideation

	Negative Problem Orientation	Rational problem Solving	Impulsiveness / Carelessness Style	Total
Adolescent Suicidal Ideation	.30*	-.22*	.23*	-.37*

*p < .0125 (Bonferroni –corrected alpha level).

Table 5. Prediction of adolescent suicidal ideation from social problem solving

Suicidal Ideation	Social	Problem	Solving		
	NPO (β)	RPS (β)	ICS (β)	R^2	*Adj.* R^2
Male	-.21***	-.19***	-.10***	.12	.12
Female	-.27***	-.19***	-.09***	.16	.15
Total	-.23***	-.19***	-.10***	.14	.14

Note: β = Standardized regression coefficient NPO= negative problem orientation RPS= rational problem solving ICS= impulsiveness / carelessness style.

*p < .05, **p < .01, ***p < .001.

Table 6. Hierarchical multiple regression analysis for the prediction of adolescent suicidal ideation in the total sample

	Step 1 (β)	Step 2 (β)	Step 3 (β)
Age	.03	.03	.02
Fathers' Job Status	-.00	.00	.01
Fathers' Education[a]	-.06**	-.05**	-.03*
Mothers' Job Status	-.01	.00	.01
Mothers' Education	.01	.00	.02
Parental Marital Status[b]	.08***	.09***	.05***
Family Income	-.01	.01	.02
CSSA Recipients	-.02	-.02	-.00
Emotional Competence		-.08***	-.00
Social Problem Solving		-.33***	-.08***
Hopelessness			.64***
F	7.53***	67.71***	316.76***
R^2	.02	.15	.47
Change in R^2		.13	.32

Note: β = Standardized regression coefficient

[a]Fathers' Education (1= Primary education or below, 2= Secondary education, 3= Tertiary education or above).

[b]Parents' Marital Status (1= intact family, 2= non-intact family, i.e. single-parent family due to death of a parent, divorce or separation).

CSSA Recipients= Comprehensive Social Security Allowance recipients.

*p < .05, **p < .01, ***p < .001.

Standard regression analysis showed that social problem solving was a significant predictor of suicidal ideation (R^2 = .14). All the three subscales were important predictors of suicidal ideation in the, total, male and female sample (see table 5). When the beta coefficients for male and female adolescents were compared (38), the coefficient of negative problem orientation with female adolescent suicidal ideation was significantly higher than that for male adolescent suicidal ideation ($z = 1.98$, $p < .05$). In the hierarchical regression analysis, when the socio-demographic characteristics were controlled, it was found that emotional competence and social problem solving accounted for an initial 13% of the variance in suicidal ideation. An additional 32% of the variance in suicidal ideation was accounted for by hopelessness. However, emotional competence was no longer a significant predictor when hopelessness was included in the equation. Overall speaking, these results indicate that hopelessness is the most important predictor of suicidal ideation, followed by social problem solving and then emotional competence (see table 6). Hypothesis 4 was thus supported. For the variation of the independent variables in relation to suicidal ideation due to differences in schools, the Wald test of Linear Mixed Model analysis indicated that it was not significant. Hence, there was no random effect of schools.

DISCUSSION

In response to the limitations in the related literature, there are several unique features of the present study. First, Chinese adolescents were recruited in this study. Second, a large sample based on Secondary 1 to Secondary 4 students was used (N = 5,557). Third, indigenously developed and validated measures of hopelessness, emotional competence, social problem solving, and suicidal ideation were used. Fourth, the relationship and relative importance of the cognitive, emotive and cognitive-behavioral correlates with adolescent suicidal ideation were examined in this study.

Result showed that parents' marital status was an important predictor of adolescent suicidal ideation. This is in line with previous finding (39). It is also consistent with the theoretical proposition that non-intact families impair the psychological well-being of adolescent members in the family. In addition, result indicated that fathers' education impacted adolescent suicidal ideation, which corroborates previous finding (40). A previous study showed that fathers with more education were found to be more confident in parenting, to be more respectful of their children and to be more warm and involved in child rearing. Since suicidal adolescents perceived their parents to be significantly more critical and less caring, educated parents who were more caring would inevitably have a better relationship with their children, which could have positive impact on the adolescents' psychological well being and lower their suicidal ideation. Both correlation and regression analysis showed that a higher level of hopelessness, a lower level of emotional competence and social problem solving was associated with a higher level of adolescent suicidal ideation. This observation is consistent with previous literature. Studies have shown that individuals with greater optimism have reduced risk for suicide ideation in the face of negative life events (2). Research has also found that adolescents who had inadequate problem solving skills were at increased risk for suicidal thoughts and behaviors (15). In addition, there are also findings showing the negative relationship of a person's emotional competence with depression (41).

The present study shows that hopelessness is the most important predictor of adolescent suicidal ideation, followed by social problem solving and then emotional competence. To explain, Chinese are comparatively more optimistic than its Western counterparts, as reflected in the Chinese sayings that "There must be a way out when the boat approaches the end of the bridge" (chuan dao qiao tou zi ran zhi). "We have nothing to fear even when the sky falls down" (tian diao xia lai dang bei gai). Conceptually, the sense of hope consists of "certainty about the future" and "future expectation". Previous studies also showed that hopelessness was significantly and inversely related to purpose in life and existential well-being (30). Hence, adolescents feeling hopeless might be really desperate, regard suicidal ideation or suicidal behavior as the only alternative available and mistakenly put their hopes on life after death (35). This explains why hopelessness is the most important predictor of adolescent suicidal ideation. Comparatively speaking, emotional competence is the least important predictor of adolescent suicidal ideation. Since Chinese culture emphasizes emotional inhibition and discouragement of expression of emotions, emotional competence might be regarded as less important by the Chinese adolescents, which in turn contributes to smaller impact on suicidal ideation.

Nevertheless, the present study showed that there were significant negative correlations between adolescent suicidal ideation and three emotional intelligence subscales, self-management of emotions, social skills and utilization of emotions, with the exception of the empathy subscale. Previous findings also indicated that there was less suicidal ideation among those high in managing others' emotions (i.e. social skills). To elaborate, research showed that adolescents who were good at managing others' emotions tended to have more social support (22). Besides, people high in social skills helped others to regulate moods in a positive direction. This behavior would lead to more intimate relationships and greater social support, which would help to protect these people from depression and suicidal ideation.

Regression analysis showed that increases in all the subscales of emotional competence, except empathy, were related to significant decrease in adolescent suicidal ideation. Interestingly, an increase in empathy was related to a significant increase in adolescent suicidal ideation. This could be explained by the fact that an empathetic person, being too sentimental and sensitive to others' emotional expression, might be easily influenced by others' positive or negative emotions. In Chinese culture, some Confucian concepts and principles similar to "empathy" are, for example, "Examine others' views by putting yourself into others' position", "Compare people's hearts with your own". They had a connotation that the person would become less self-centered and more other-centered. The self was suppressed in order to enter others' hearts to understand their feelings and viewpoint. Since Chinese had strong social orientation and were attentive and sensitive to others' needs, they were usually too emotionally involved in others' sorrow and misery. Being too emotionally involved might increase personal burden and might not be healthy for individual functioning. Hence, an adolescent might be more prone to developing suicidal ideation when he was empathetic with others' feelings, especially negative emotions.

Of the four subscales, social skills subscale was not an important predictor of female adolescent suicidal ideation. Traditionally, Chinese females have been described as affectionate, charming, emotional, gentle, kind and warm. They might be too familiar with complimenting and helping others develop positive emotions. This type of altruistic satisfaction would not be strong enough to protect them against suicidal ideation. Both correlation and regression analysis showed that self management of emotions was strongly related to, and an important predictor of adolescent suicidal ideation. A person's awareness, understanding and regulation of his own emotions were important in decreasing his suicidal ideation. This is consistent with previous research on the relationship between emotion regulation, emotion expression and depression (18). Although previous literature also revealed that affect dysregulation had been associated with adolescent suicidal behavior, the present study was pioneering in identifying self management of emotions as an important predictor of adolescent suicidal ideation.

Although there were significant negative correlations between adolescent suicidal ideation and all three subscales of social problem solving, negative problem orientation was the subscale most strongly related to and the most important predictor of adolescent suicidal ideation. This observation was consistent with the previous finding that negative problem orientation was most highly correlated with suicidal risk, followed by an avoidance or impulsive problem-solving style (42). A Hong Kong study also showed that negative problem orientation had a stronger relationship with measures of family functioning than did impulsiveness / carelessness style (43). Adolescents with a negative problem orientation tended to view a problem as a significant "threat" to well-being, have self-blame for problems, have low confidence in solving problems successfully, believe that problems could hardly be solved and be emotionally sensitive to problems. Since they believed that the problems were difficult to be solved and there were no other alternatives, they might develop suicidal ideation and think that suicide was the only way out.

Moreover, adolescents who were impulsive might fare even worse as they tended to avoid problems, delay solving problems for as long as possible, wait for problems to resolve themselves, and attempt to shift responsibility for solving his problems to others. Hwang (44) found that besides mobilization of personal resources, seeking help from social resources and appealing to supernatural power, Chinese people also tended to adopt the philosophy of doing nothing or avoidance as a coping strategy when facing problems. Furthermore, adolescents with ineffective rational problem solving skills lacked the abilities and skills to solve the problems. When the adolescents lacked rational problem solving skills and adopted avoidance strategy, they might be overwhelmed by the problems, thus creating stress and suicidal ideation.

Regression analysis showed that the beta coefficient of negative problem orientation with female adolescent suicidal ideation was significantly higher than that for male adolescent suicidal ideation. Since females had more negative problem orientations, greater avoidance tendencies and less ability to generate alternative solutions, they tended to turn to suicidal ideation more easily, while males might resort to alternative ways of coping even though they had a negative problem orientation. There is a need to further investigate why negative problem orientation is more significantly related to female suicidal ideation than male suicidal ideation.

From the above discussion, it can be shown that the results are consistent with the cognitive, emotive and cognitive-behavioral theories that postulate hopelessness, emotional competence and social problem solving have impacts on suicidal ideation. Although hopelessness is the most important predictor of suicidal ideation, social problem solving and emotional competence should also be considered as the key building blocks in theoretical models for adolescent suicidal ideation. This adds evidence to the cognitive, emotive and cognitive-behavioral models in explaining adolescent suicidal ideation in the Chinese context. However, emotional competence has the least impact on adolescent suicidal ideation.

Practically speaking, it is recommended to use an integrative cognitive-emotive-behavioral approach to reduce adolescent suicidal ideation. Since the cognitive correlate, hopelessness, is positively related to adolescent suicidal ideation, it is important to cultivate the sense of hope in adolescents. A study has shown that increasing one's positive future expectations, identifying and pursuing one's life goals and plans, could reduce suicide risk (45). Workshops and programs can be conducted to help adolescents build up hope and future expectations, develop positive attitudes to exploring possible options in life and recognize their own capabilities in goal achievement. Some adventure-based counseling, i.e. implementation and debriefing of adventure activities to enhance self-understanding, coping with adversity and interpersonal co-operation, can be introduced so that adolescents can learn to persevere in face of hardship.

Besides, it is important to enhance emotional competence, the emotive correlate, among adolescents. Buckley, Storino and Saarni (46) reported that mastery of the skills of emotional competence was contributive to positive youth development. Specifically, groups and workshops could be organized for adolescents to understand and regulate their own emotions and manage others' emotions, as well as make effective use of emotions. Although there are some local programs, e.g. "Positive Adolescent Training through Holistic Social Programs" (P.A.T.H.S.) (47-50), to develop students' awareness of their emotions and proper emotional expression, there is a lack of emphasis on social skills and the utilization of emotions, which are significant predictors of adolescent suicidal ideation, in these programs. Since the Chinese adolescents were socialized to suppress their emotions and an 'ideal' person was characterized by self-constraint and control of emotions in Chinese societies, practitioners should also take note of this unique problem of Chinese people regarding emotional expression and possible cultural barrier in conducting such workshops and programs.

Since the cognitive-behavioral component, social problem solving, is negatively related to suicidal ideation, it is important to enhance rational problem solving skills, decrease negative problem orientation and impulsiveness / carelessness style among adolescents. A local study showed that cognitive-behavioral group intervention, introducing rational thinking and coping skills, was effective in helping persons at risk of developing mental health problems in Hong Kong (51). The P.A.T.H.S. (52-55), which included problem solving and resilience training, was found to be effective in reducing the negative behaviors of secondary school students. However, an integrative intervention approach comprising all the cognitive, emotive and behavioral elements is recommended.

Because adolescent social problem solving abilities were not strongly encouraged in Chinese families, it might be difficult for adolescents to adapt to learning such skills. Practitioners should try to change the adolescents from negative coping and avoidance to active coping attitudes when facing problems. Workshops and programs could be held to teach the adolescents rational problem solving skills such as problem definition and formulation, generation of alternative solutions, decision making, solution implementation and verification, as well as to cultivate a positive problem orientation and to introduce active coping strategies.

It is noteworthy that there are several limitations of the present study. First, schools have been approached through agencies providing school social work service, and the resulting samples thus represent convenience samples. In particular, generalizing the present findings to the broader secondary school population should proceed with caution. Second, as self-report questionnaires were used, the information collected was based on the adolescent informants only. If resource permits, the use of multiple informants would give a clearer picture of the problem area. Third, the present research predominately used quantitative methodology. One disadvantage of this methodology is that it cannot explore the subjective experiences of adolescents. Another drawback is that it is less process-oriented and difficult to apply the generalized data to individual cases. Fourth, besides the correlates utilized in this study, other cognitive, emotive and cognitive-behavioral indicators should also be used in future. Fifth, the use of a cross-sectional design means that it is not possible to claim a causal relationship between the antecedents and adolescent suicidal ideation. There may in fact be a bi-directional relationship between the variables, or a third variable may be present. Hence, a longitudinal research design can be used in future studies. Despite these limitations, the present study highlights the importance of cognitive, emotive, and cognitive-behavioral factors in adolescent suicidal ideation.

REFERENCES

[1] Rush AJ, Beck AT. Cognitive therapy of depression and suicide. Am J Psychother 1978;32(2):201-19.
[2] Gençöz F, Vatan S, Walker R, Lester D. A brief research note: Helplessness, hopelessness, and haplessness as predictors of suicidal ideation: a cross-cultural study. Omega 2008;57(3):315-8.
[3] Stewart SM, Kennard BD, Lee PWH, Mayes T, Hughes C, Emslie G. Hopelessness and suicidal ideation among adolescents in two cultures. J Child Psychol Psychiatry 2005;46(4):364-72.
[4] Rucklidge JJ. Psychosocial functioning of adolescents with and without paediatric bipolar disorder. J Affect Disord 2006;91(2-3):181-8.
[5] Bentley KW. Predictors of suicide ideation, depression, and hopelessness in high school and college students. US: ProQuest InformationLearning, 1999:1841.
[6] Goleman D. Emotional intelligence: Why it can matter more than IQ. London: Bloomsbury, 1996.
[7] Tamás Z, Kovacs M, Gentzler AL, Tepper P, Gádoros J, Kiss E, et al. The relations of temperament and emotion self-regulation with suicidal behaviors in a clinical sample of depressed children in Hungary. J Abnorm Child Psychol 2007;35(4):640-52.
[8] Sheeber L, Allen N, Davis B, Sorensen E. Regulation of negative affect during mother¡Vchild problem-solving interactions: adolescent depressive status and family processes. J Abnorm Child Psychol 2000;28(5):467-79.
[9] Thayer JF, Rossy LA, Ruiz-Padial E, Johnsen BH. Gender differences in the relationship between emotional regulation and depressive symptoms. Cognit Ther Res 2003;27(3):349-64.
[10] Zhang JS, Shen LX, Gao N. The revision and application of the revision of the Early Adolescent Temperament Questionnaire. Chinese Ment Health J 2008;22(6):439-43.
[11] Camras LA, Ribordy S, Hill J, Martino S, Sachs V, Spaccarelli S, Stefani R. Maternal facial behavior and the recognition and production of emotional expression by maltreated and nonmaltreated children. Dev Psychol 1990;26(2):304-12.
[12] D'Zurilla TJ, Maydeu-Olivares A. Conceptual and methodological issues in social problem-solving assessment. Behav Ther 1995;26(3):409-32.
[13] D'Zurilla TJ, Nezu AM, Maydeu-Olivares A. Manual for the Social Problem-Solving Inventory-Revised (SPSI-R). New York: Multi-Health System, 1996.
[14] Rudd MD. The suicidal mode: a cognitive-behavioral model of suicidality. Suicide Life Threat Behav 2000;30(1):18-33.
[15] Eskin M, Ertekin K, Dereboy C, Demirkiran F. Risk factors for and protective factors against adolescent suicidal behavior in Turkey. Crisis 2007;28(3):131-9.
[16] Kingsbury S, Hawton K, Steinhardt K, James A. Do adolescents who take overdoses have specific psychological characteristics? A comparative study with psychiatric and community controls. J Am Acad Child Adolesc Psychiatry 1999;38(9):1125-31.
[17] Kashden J, Fremouw WJ, Callahan TS, Franzen MD. Impulsivity in suicidal and nonsuicidal adolescents. J Abnorm Child Psychol 1993;21(3):339-53.
[18] Calvete E, Cardeñoso O. Gender differences in cognitive vulnerability to depression and behavior problems in adolescents. J Abnorm Child Psychol 2005;33(2):179-92.

[19] Poon W-T, Lau S. Coping with failure: relationship with self-concept discrepancy and attributional style. J Soc Psychol 1999;139(5): 639-53.
[20] Siu AM-H. Interpersonal competence, family functioning, and parent-adolescent conflicts. US: ProQuest Information Learning, 2003:3733.
[21] Williams JMG, Pollock LR. Factors mediating suicidal behaviour: their utility in primary and secondary prevention. J Ment Health 1993;2(1):3-26.
[22] Ciarrochi J, Scott G, Deane FP, Heaven PCL. Relations between social and emotional competence and mental health: a construct validation study. Pers Individ Diff 2003;35(8):1947-63.
[23] Ceperich SRD. Coping interventions for high school-based suicide prevention. US: ProQuest Information Learning, 1997.
[24] Yang B, Clum GA. Life stress, social support, and problem-solving skills predictive of depressive symptoms, hopelessness, and suicide ideation in an Asian student population: a test of a model. Suicide Life Threat Behav 1994;24(2):127-39.
[25] Edwards MJ, Holden RR. Coping, meaning in life, and suicidal manifestations: examining gender differences. J Clin Psychol 2003;59(10):1133-50.
[26] Silviken A, Kvernmo S. Suicide attempts among indigenous Sami adolescents and majority peers in Arctic Norway: prevalence and associated risk factors. J Adolescence 2007;30(4):613-26.
[27] Goodman E. The role of socioeconomic status gradients in explaining differences in US adolescents' health. Am J Public Health 1999;89(10):1522-8.
[28] Cheung YB, Law CK, Chan B, Liu KY, Yip PSF. Suicidal ideation and suicidal attempts in a population-based study of Chinese people: risk attributable to hopelessness, depression, and social factors. J Affect Disord 2006;90(2-3):193-9.
[29] Bond MH. The handbook of Chinese psychology. New York: Oxford University Press, 1996.
[30] Beck AT, Weissman A, Lester D, Trexler L. The measurement of pessimism: The Hopelessness Scale. J Consult Clin Psychol 1974;42(6):861-5.
[31] Shek DTL. Measurement of pessimism in Chinese adolescents: the Chinese Hopelessness Scale. Soc Behav Pers 1993;21(2):107-119.
[32] Shek DTL, Lee TY. Hopelessness in Chinese adolescents in Hong Kong. In: Merrick J, Zalsman G, eds. Suicidal behavior in adolescence: An international perspective. London: Freund, 2005:105-18.
[33] Chan DW. Dimensions of emotional intelligence and their relationships with social coping among gifted adolescents in Hong Kong. J. Youth Adolescence 2003;32(6):409-18.
[34] Schutte NS, Malouff JM, Hall LE, Haggerty DJ, Cooper JT, Golden CJ, Dornheim L. Development and validation of a measure of emotional intelligence. Pers Individ Diff 1998;25(2):167-77.
[35] Siu AMH, Shek DTL. The Chinese version of the social problem-solving inventory: some initial results on reliability and validity. J Clin Psychol 2005;61(3):347-60.
[36] Tse WL, Bagley C. Suicidal behavior, bereavement and death education in Chinese adolescents. Aldershot: Ashgate, 2002.
[37] Linden M. Posttraumatic embitterment disorder and wisdom therapy. J Cogn Psychol 2008;22(1):4-14.
[38] Cohen J, Cohen P. Applied multiple regression. Correlation analysis for the behavioral sciences. Mahwah, NJ: Lawrence Erlbaum, 1983.
[39] Herrara A, Dahlblom K, Dahlgren L, Kullgren J. Pathways to suicidal behavior among adolescent girls in Nicaragua. Soc Sci Med 2006;62(4):805-14.
[40] Zeng Q. An exploratory study of child temperament and parenting: a Chinese perspective. US: ProQuest Information Learning, 1999:0860.
[41] Znoj HJ, Lude P. Regulation of emotion and psychological symptoms in people with spinal cord injury. Swiss J Psychol 2002;61(4):203-10.
[42] Reinecke MA, DuBois DL, Schultz TM. Social problem solving, mood, and suicidality among inpatient adolescents. Cognit Ther Res 2001;25(6):743-56.
[43] Siu AMH, Shek DTL. Relations between social problem solving and indicators of interpersonal and family well-being among Chinese adolescents in Hong Kong. Soc Indic Res 2005;71(1):517-39.
[44] Hwang KK. The patterns of coping strategies in a Chinese society. Acta Psychol Taiwanica 1997;19:61-73.

[45] O'Connor RC, Connery H, Cheyne, W.M. Hopelessness: the role of depression, future directed thinking and cognitive vulnerability. Psychol Health Med 2000;5(2):155-61.
[46] Buckley M, Storino M, Saarni C. Promoting emotional competence in children and adolescents: implications for school psychologists. Sch Psychol Q 2003;18(2):177-91.
[47] Shek DTL, Sun RCF. Helping adolescents with greater psychosocial needs: evaluation of a positive youth development program. ScientificWorldJournal 2008;8:575-85.
[48] Shek DTL. Effectiveness of the Tier 1 Program of the Project P.A.T.H.S.: findings based on the first 2 years of program implementation. ScientificWorldJournal 2009;9:539-47.
[49] Shek DTL, Ma HK. Evaluation of Project P.A.T.H.S. (Secondary 1 Program) by the program implementers: findings based on the full implementation phase. ScientificWorldJournal 2008;8: 492-501.
[50] Shek DTL, Sun RCF, Chan CWY. Evaluation of Project P.A.T.H.S. (Secondary 2 Program) by the program participants: findings based on the experimental implementation phase. Scientific World Journal 2008;8:526-35.
[51] Wong DFK, Sun SYK, Tse J, Wong F. Evaluating the outcomes of a cognitive-behavioral group intervention model for persons at risk of developing mental health problems in Hong Kong: a pretest-posttest study. Res Soc Work Pract 2002;12(4):534-45.
[52] Shek DTL, Ng CSM. Secondary 1 Program of Project P.A.T.H.A.: process evaluation based on the co-walker scheme. ScientificWorldJournal 2009;9:704-14.
[53] Shek DTL. Evaluation of the Tier 1 Program of Project P.A.T.H.S.: secondary data analyses of conclusions drawn by the program implementers. ScientificWorldJournal 2008;8:22-34.
[54] Shek DTL. Effectiveness of the Tier 1 Program of Project P.A.T.H.S.: findings based on the first 2 years of program implementation. ScientificWorldJournal 2009;9:539-47.
[55] Shek DTL, Ma HK. Editorial: evaluation of the Project P.A.T.H.S. in Hong Kong: are the findings replicable across different populations? ScientificWorldJournal 2010;10:178–81.

ACKNOWLEDGMENTS

In: Adolescence and Behavior Issues in a Chinese Context ISBN: 978-1-62618-614-9
Editors: DTL Shek, RCF Sun and Joav Merrick

Chapter 13

ABOUT THE EDITORS

Daniel TL Shek, PhD, FHKPS, BBS, JP, is Chair Professor of Applied Social Sciences, Department of Applied Social Sciences, Hong Kong Polytechnic University, Hunghom, Hong Kong, PRC, Advisory Professor of East China Normal University and Honorary Professor of Kiang Wu Nursing College of Macau. He is Chief Editor of *Journal of Youth Studies*, Consulting Editor of *Journal of Clinical Psychology*, international consultant of *American Journal of Family Therapy*, and editorial board member of *Social Indicators Research, International Journal of Adolescent Medicine and Health, The Scientific World Journal (Child Health and Human Development and Holistic Health and Medicine domains), Asian Journal of Counseling, International Journal of Disability and Human Development,* and *Bentham Open Family Studies Journal*. He has served in many government advisory bodies, including the Action Committee against Narcotics, Commission on Youth, Fight Crime Committee and Family Council. He has published numerous books, book chapters and more than 300 scientific articles in international refereed journals. E-mail: daniel.shek@polyu.edu.hk

Rachel CF Sun, PhD, is assistant professor at the Faculty of Education, The University of Hong Kong, Hong Kong, PRC. She teaches in the areas of psychology of teaching and learning, and child and adolescent development. Her research areas include academic achievement motivation, student misbehavior, school satisfaction, life satisfaction, positive youth development, adolescent suicidal ideation and psychological health. She is a co-principal investigator of a huge and pioneering positive youth development project in Hong Kong. She is an Executive Committee member of the Society of Boys' Centres, and a member of the Editorial Board of *Research on Social Work Practice*. E-mail: rachels@hku.hk

Joav Merrick, MD, MMedSci, DMSc, is professor of pediatrics, child health and human development affiliated with Kentucky Children's Hospital, University of Kentucky, Lexington, United States and the Division of Pediatrics, Hadassah Hebrew University Medical Centers, Mt Scopus Campus, Jerusalem, Israel, the medical director of the Health Services, Division for Intellectual and Developmental Disabilities, Ministry of Social Affairs and Social Services, Jerusalem, the founder and director of the National Institute of Child Health and Human Development in Israel. Numerous publications in the field of pediatrics, child health and human development, rehabilitation, intellectual disability, disability, health, welfare, abuse, advocacy, quality of life and prevention. Received the Peter Sabroe Child Award for outstanding work on behalf of Danish Children in 1985 and the International LEGO-Prize ("The Children's Nobel Prize") for an extraordinary contribution towards improvement in child welfare and well-being in 1987. E-mail: jmerrick@zahav.net.il

In: Adolescence and Behavior Issues in a Chinese Context ISBN: 978-1-62618-614-9
Editors: DTL Shek, RCF Sun and Joav Merrick

Chapter 14

About the Department of Applied Social Sciences, the Hong Kong Polytechnic University

The Department of Applied Social Sciences (APSS) of The Hong Kong Polytechnic University is one of the largest and most vibrant centres in the region dedicated to the education and training of professional social workers, social policy and welfare administrators, psychologists and counselors in Hong Kong.

The Department started as the Institute of Social Work Training in 1973. It joined the Hong Kong Polytechnic in 1977 and became its School of Social Work. The School was eventually renamed the Department of Applied Social Sciences. APSS celebrated its 35th anniversary in the academic year of 2007/08. Currently there are 93 full-time academics, over 80 research/project staff, 20 fieldwork supervisors and 34 colleagues in other categories, including administrative and supporting personnel.

The Department has six thriving Research Centres: Centre for Social Policy Studies, China Research and Development Network, Network for Health and Welfare Studies, Professional Practice and Assessment Centre, Centre for Third Sector Studies, and the Manulife Centre for Children with Specific Learning Disabilities, providing platforms for collaborative research and practice projects with government departments and NGOs.

The Department of Applied Social Sciences offers taught programs in the fields of Social Work, Social Policy and Administration, Counseling, and Applied Psychology, as well as research degrees at MPhil and PhD levels. In 2008/09, APSS offered some 20 Programs for Higher Diploma, Degree, Postgraduate, MPhil and PhD students. There are currently about 1,500 students enrolled in the various APSS programs and we have graduated more than 14,000 students over the years.

In the past decade, the Department has successfully expanded into the Chinese mainland. The Department currently offers a MSW(China) Program in collaboration with Peking University and a Joint PolyU-PekingU Social Work Research Centre has been established to foster research in social work and social policy.

Contact

Professor Daniel TL Shek, PhD, FHKPS, BBS, JP
Chair Professor of Applied Social Sciences
Department of Applied Social Sciences
The Hong Kong Polytechnic University
Hunghom, Hong Kong
E-mail: daniel.shek@polyu.edu.hk

In: Adolescence and Behavior Issues in a Chinese Context
Editors: DTL Shek, RCF Sun and Joav Merrick
ISBN: 978-1-62618-614-9

Chapter 15

ABOUT THE NATIONAL INSTITUTE OF CHILD HEALTH AND HUMAN DEVELOPMENT IN ISRAEL

The National Institute of Child Health and Human Development (NICHD) in Israel was established in 1998 as a virtual institute under the auspicies of the Medical Director, Ministry of Social Affairs and Social Services in order to function as the research arm for the Office of the Medical Director. In 1998 the National Council for Child Health and Pediatrics, Ministry of Health and in 1999 the Director General and Deputy Director General of the Ministry of Health endorsed the establishment of the NICHD. In 2011 the NICHD became affiliated with the Division of Pediatrics, Hadassah Hebrew University Medical Center, Mt Scopus Campus in Jerusalem.

MISSION

The mission of a National Institute for Child Health and Human Development in Israel is to provide an academic focal point for the scholarly interdisciplinary study of child life, health, public health, welfare, disability, rehabilitation, intellectual disability and related aspects of human development. This mission includes research, teaching, clinical work, information and public service activities in the field of child health and human development.

SERVICE AND ACADEMIC ACTIVITIES

Over the years many activities became focused in the south of Israel due to collaboration with various professionals at the Faculty of Health Sciences (FOHS) at the Ben Gurion University of the Negev (BGU). Since 2000 an affiliation with the Zusman Child Development Center at the Pediatric Division of Soroka University Medical Center has resulted in collaboration around the establishment of the Down Syndrome Clinic at that center. In 2002 a full course on "Disability" was established at the Recanati School for Allied Professions in the Community, FOHS, BGU and in 2005 collaboration was started with the Primary Care Unit of the faculty and disability became part of the master of public health course on "Children and society". In the academic year 2005-2006 a one semester course on "Aging with disability" was started as part of the master of science program in gerontology in our collaboration with the Center for Multidisciplinary Research in Aging. In 2010 collaborations with the Division of Pediatrics, Hadassah Hebrew University Medical Center, Jerusalem, Israel around the National Down Syndrome Center and teaching students and residents about intellectual and developmental disabilities as part of their training at this campus.

RESEARCH ACTIVITIES

The affiliated staff have over the years published work from projects and research activities in this national and international collaboration. In the year 2000 the International Journal of Adolescent Medicine and Health and in 2005 the International Journal on Disability and Human Development of De Gruyter Publishing House (Berlin and New York) were affiliated with the National Institute of Child Health and Human Development. From 2008 also the International Journal of Child Health and Human Development (Nova Science, New York), the International Journal of Child and Adolescent Health (Nova Science) and the Journal of Pain Management (Nova Science) affiliated and from 2009 the International Public Health Journal (Nova Science) and Journal of Alternative Medicine Research (Nova Science). All peer-reviewed international journals.

NATIONAL COLLABORATIONS

Nationally the NICHD works in collaboration with the Faculty of Health Sciences, Ben Gurion University of the Negev; Department of Physical Therapy, Sackler School of Medicine, Tel Aviv University; Autism Center, Assaf HaRofeh Medical Center; National Rett and PKU Centers at Chaim Sheba Medical Center, Tel HaShomer; Department of Physiotherapy, Haifa University; Department of Education, Bar Ilan University, Ramat Gan, Faculty of Social Sciences and Health Sciences; College of Judea and Samaria in Ariel and in 2011 affiliation with Center for Pediatric Chronic Diseases and National Center for Down Syndrome, Department of Pediatrics, Hadassah Hebrew University Medical Center, Mount Scopus Campus, Jerusalem.

INTERNATIONAL COLLABORATIONS

Internationally with the Department of Disability and Human Development, College of Applied Health Sciences, University of Illinois at Chicago; Strong Center for Developmental Disabilities, Golisano Children's Hospital at Strong, University of Rochester School of Medicine and Dentistry, New York; Centre on Intellectual Disabilities, University of Albany, New York; Centre for Chronic Disease Prevention and Control, Health Canada, Ottawa; Chandler Medical Center and Children's Hospital, Kentucky Children's Hospital, Section of Adolescent Medicine, University of Kentucky, Lexington; Chronic Disease Prevention and Control Research Center, Baylor College of Medicine, Houston, Texas; Division of Neuroscience, Department of Psychiatry, Columbia University, New York; Institute for the

Study of Disadvantage and Disability, Atlanta; Center for Autism and Related Disorders, Department Psychiatry, Children's Hospital Boston, Boston; Department of Paediatrics, Child Health and Adolescent Medicine, Children's Hospital at Westmead, Westmead, Australia; International Centre for the Study of Occupational and Mental Health, Düsseldorf, Germany; Centre for Advanced Studies in Nursing, Department of General Practice and Primary Care, University of Aberdeen, Aberdeen, United Kingdom; Quality of Life Research Center, Copenhagen, Denmark; Nordic School of Public Health, Gottenburg, Sweden, Scandinavian Institute of Quality of Working Life, Oslo, Norway; The Department of Applied Social Sciences (APSS) of The Hong Kong Polytechnic University Hong Kong.

TARGETS

Our focus is on research, international collaborations, clinical work, teaching and policy in health, disability and human development and to establish the NICHD as a permanent institute at one of the residential care centers for persons with intellectual disability in Israel in order to conduct model research and together with the four university schools of public health/medicine in Israel establish a national master and doctoral program in disability and human development at the institute to secure the next generation of professionals working in this often non-prestigious/low-status field of work.

Contact

Joav Merrick, MD, DMSc

Professor of Pediatrics, Child Health and Human Development

Medical Director, Health Services, Division for Intellectual and Developmental Disabilities, Ministry of Social Affairs and Social Services, POB 1260, IL-91012 Jerusalem, Israel.

E-mail: jmerrick@zahav.net.il

In: Adolescence and Behavior Issues in a Chinese Context ISBN: 978-1-62618-614-9
Editors: DTL Shek, RCF Sun and Joav Merrick

Chapter 16

About the Book Series "Pediatrics, Child and Adolescent Health"

Pediatrics, child and adolescent health is a book series with publications from a multidisciplinary group of researchers, practitioners and clinicians for an international professional forum interested in the broad spectrum of pediatric medicine, child health, adolescent health and human development.

- Merrick J, ed. Child and adolescent health yearbook 2011. New York: Nova Science, 2012.
- Merrick J, ed. Child and adolescent health yearbook 2012. New York: Nova Science, 2012.
- Roach RR, Greydanus DE, Patel DR, Homnick DN, Merrick J, eds. Tropical pediatrics: A public health concern of international proportions. New York: Nova Science, 2012.
- Merrick J, ed. Child health and human development yearbook 2011. New York: Nova Science, 2012.
- Merrick J, ed. Child health and human development yearbook 2012. New York: Nova Science, 2012.
- Shek DTL, Sun RCF, Merrick J, eds. Developmental issues in Chinese adolescents. New York: Nova Science, 2012.
- Shek DTL, Sun RCF, Merrick J, eds. Positive youth development: Theory, research and application. New York: Nova Science, 2012.
- Zachor DA, Merrick J, eds. Understanding autism spectrum disorder: Current research aspects. New York: Nova Science, 2012.
- Ma HK, Shek DTL, Merrick J, eds. Positive youth development: A new school curriculum to tackle adolescent developmental issues. New York: Nova Science, 2012.
- Wood D, Reiss JG, Ferris ME, Edwards LR, Merrick J, eds. Transition from pediatric to adult medical care. New York: Nova Science, 2012.

Contact

Professor Joav Merrick, MD, MMedSci, DMSc
Medical Director, Medical Services
Division for Intellectual and Developmental Disabilities
Ministry of Social Affairs and Social Services
POBox 1260
IL-91012 Jerusalem, Israel
E-mail: jmerrick@zahav.net.il

INDEX

D

E

F

G

H

I

Q

R

S

T

U

V

W

Y